1994

# Atlas of
# Ovarian Tumors

# Atlas of Ovarian Tumors

**Liane Deligdisch, M.D.**
Professor of Pathology
Professor of Obstetrics, Gynecology
and Reproductive Science
Director, Division of Gynecologic Pathology
Department of Pathology
The Mount Sinai Medical Center
New York, New York

**Albert Altchek, M.D.**
Clinical Professor of Obstetrics,
Gynecology and Reproductive Science
The Mount Sinai Medical Center
New York, New York

**Carmel J. Cohen, M.D.**
Professor of Obstetrics,
Gynecology and Reproductive Science
Director, Division of Gynecological Oncology
Vice-Chairman, Department of Obstetrics/Gynecology
The Mount Sinai Medical Center
New York, New York

**Igaku-Shoin   New York • Tokyo**

*To the memory of Elka, Annie, Rachel, and the
many other women who have died of ovarian cancer.*

Published and distributed by

IGAKU-SHOIN Medical Publishers, Inc.
One Madison Avenue, New York, N.Y. 10010

IGAKU-SHOIN Ltd.,
5-24-3 Hongo, Bunkyo-ku, Tokyo 113-91

**Library of Congress Cataloging-in-Publication Data**

Deligdisch, Liane.
    Atlas of ovarian tumors / Liane Deligdisch, Albert Altchek,
Carmel J. Cohen.
        p.        cm.
    Includes bibliographical references and index.
    1. Ovaries—Tumors—Atlases.   I. Altchek, Albert,
1925–  .  II. Cohen, Carmel J.  III. Title.
    [DNLM: 1. Ovarian Neoplasms—atlases.   WP 17 D353a   1994]
RC280.08045  1994
616.99'265—dc20
DNLM/DLC
for Library of Congress                         93-27160
                                                    CIP

ISBN: 0-89640-240-1 (New York)
ISBN: 4-260-14240-2 (Tokyo)

Printed and bound in the U.S.A.

10 9 8 7 6 5 4 3 2 1

# Preface

Despite a recent proliferation of excellent textbooks of gynecologic oncology and ovarian cancer, there has been a noticeable absence of an atlas of ovarian tumors.

There is no standard current atlas! The standard reference had been the classic *Tumors of the Ovary and Maldeveloped Gonads* by Robert E. Scully of Harvard Medical School. It was one of the fascicles of the *Atlas of Tumor Pathology* series published by the Armed Forces Institute of Pathology, Washington, D.C. It had been published in 1979 (second series, fascicle 16) and is now out of print. The series was published in different segments, at different times, and by different authors.

There is a need for a new atlas of ovarian tumors. Concepts and teaching methods change with time. Since fresh gross specimens and histologic slides are seen in color and since interpreting images has a strong subjective aspect, quality color reproduction is essential. The technology of color printing has now achieved perfection. An atlas is required by the student and experienced pathologist as a review, update, and reference.

Of equal and perhaps of even more importance, an atlas is needed to help the clinician (1) rapidly understand the pathologic appearance of a lesion by seeing pictures rather than by tediously trying to visualize a verbal description and (2) communicate better with the pathologist by understanding the pathologist's terminology and what the pathologist is describing. Thus, the clinician should be able to better comprehend the brief, terse report on a frozen section during the anxious time of surgery as well as the final complete report.

This atlas is a new book, done at one time with a fresh contemporary viewpoint, with color illustrations magnificently printed on quality paper.

Aside from directly contributing to patient care, this atlas by virtue of its clinical orientation can serve as a basic framework for research and a springboard for investigative pathology. It should therefore become a dialogue between the pathologist and clinician.

Albert Altchek, M.D.

# Foreword

The *Atlas of Ovarian Tumors* is a well-written and illustrated treatise on tumors of the ovary. It is written by three outstanding physicians (Drs. Liane Deligdisch, A. Altchek, and C. J. Cohen), each providing their individual expertise to this outstanding *Atlas*.

The *Atlas* is designed to offer both practicing gynecologists and pathologists images and text to illustrate the most common and some less common ovarian neoplasms. Special emphasis is directed to early diagnosis and particularly to histologic characteristics of early, preinvasive ovarian neoplasms. One chapter of great interest includes original research based on computerized image analysis of ovarian intraepithelial neoplasia (OIN) and morphometric studies of tissue obtained by second-look operations revealing changes associated with the use of anticancer chemotherapy.

There are no weaknesses in this wonderfully written and designed *Atlas*. It will be helpful to pathologists and clinicians in diagnosing ovarian tumors. The *Atlas* is especially valuable in supplying background for diagnosing ovarian tumors in early stages.

The chapter introducing the *Atlas* is the most thorough discussion of all aspects of ovarian tumors that I have ever read. It is a concise, accurate, and up-to-date review of the essentials in studying ovarian tumors. It merits the designation of "the ABC's of ovarian tumors for the clinician, pathologist, students, and family practitioners." This *Atlas* serves both the needs of continuing medical education and those seeking to deliver optimal health care. The material is presented in a readable manner without being superficial. The authors have achieved this and more. They have brought the art and science of ovarian tumors together for the benefit of the patient and have lightened the work of the busy clinician.

The *Atlas* is a book of facts, useful for a range of physicians. Medical students will appreciate the thorough but uncluttered presentation of the where, why, and how of detection, diagnosis, and management. For clinicians, the recommendations for diagnostic procedures and guidelines for studying patients suspected of having ovarian cancers will be appreciated. The treatment methods outlined contain valuable information for all physicians who treat women. The resident will find new understanding about facts already known, amplified by liberal background information. The gynecologic oncologist will find a well-organized base for building additional knowledge of this disease. It provides the nongynecologic physician with a ready-reference source.

Unlike so many *Atlases,* this one has gross and microphotographs that are of superior technical and esthetic quality. It is a joy to study them.

This *Atlas* is long overdue. It will contribute significantly toward a better knowledge of ovarian tumors by all physicians who give health care to women. This knowledge is of great importance, for the symptoms of ovarian tumors are protean and may simulate those more typical of other abdominal organ systems. An awareness of the subject will speed the discovery of ovarian tumors at an earlier stage.

Since I have a lifelong interest in this subject, I read the *Atlas* carefully and congratulate the authors on a job well done. It will long remain a hallmark publication.

Hugh R. K. Barber, M.D.

# Contributors

**Vladimir Bychkov, M.D.**
Associate Professor of Pathology
Mount Sinai School of Medicine
New York, New York

and

Director, Department of Pathology
Elmhurst Hospital Center
Queens, New York

**Tamara Kalir, M.D., Ph.D.**
Assistant Professor of Pathology
The Mount Sinai Medical Center
Mount Sinai School of Medicine
New York, New York

# Acknowledgment

The authors want to thank Ms. Fortune Uy for preparing the manuscript.

# Contents

# 1

## Clinical Aspects
### DIAGNOSIS AND MANAGEMENT

# 1

# General Considerations

*Albert Altchek, M.D.*

The American Cancer Society has estimated that in 1993, there would be 22,000 new cases of ovarian cancer and 13,300 deaths from it.[1] "It is estimated that one of every 70 women will develop ovarian cancer during her lifetime."[2] New cases of cervical cancer in 1993 were estimated at 13,500, with 4400 deaths; new cases of uterine corpus cancer were estimated at 31,000, with 5700 deaths. Therefore, ovarian cancer, although second in incidence of gynecologic cancer, causes more deaths than all other gynecologic cancers combined.[1]

Ovarian cancer represents 4% of all cancer cases.[2] It is the sixth most common cancer in women (21,000 new cases per year), being preceded by breast cancer (180,000), colon and rectal cancer (77,000), lung cancer (66,000), uterine cancer (45,500), and lymphoma (21,200) (nonmelanoma skin cancer and carcinoma in situ are excluded). Ovarian cancer is tied with pancreatic cancer as the fourth most common cause of cancer death in women (13,000 deaths per year), being preceded by cancer of the lung (53,000), breast (46,000), and colon and rectum (29,400).[2]

Most ovarian cancers (about 85%) are common epithelial serous and mucinous cystadenocarcinomas.[2] The 5-year survival rate for ovarian cancer is 39%, while that for cervical cancer is 66% and that for uterine corpus cancer, 83%.

The reason for the dismal prognosis for ovarian cancer is that most cases (about 77%) are discovered with advanced disease; it is the most frequent late-discovered cancer.[2] The 5-year survival rate for local disease with cancer confined to the ovary is 87%, with local cervical disease it is 88%, and with local corpus disease it is 93%. With regional spread, the 5-year survival rate drops for all, but, in addition, the drop is relatively greater for ovarian cancer, with a 5-year survival of 39%, while the drop for cervical cancer is to 52%, and that for corpus cancer, to 70%. For distant spread, the 5-year survival rate for ovarian cancer is 19%; for cervical cancer, 14%; and for corpus cancer, 27%.

Despite advances in knowledge, surgical resection and debulking, second-look surgery, and chemotherapy, survival of patients with ovarian cancer (meaning advanced cancer) has not improved dramatically, with the death rate relatively stable from 1960 to 1989.[1] Only 15 to 20% of advanced ovarian cancer cases are curable. Even platinum-based chemotherapy, which has improved response and duration remissions, has only given a modest improvement in overall survival.[3A]

In 1958 in the United States, there were 7579 deaths from ovarian cancer.[2] In 1988, the deaths had increased to 12,397. Although there were more deaths, the death rate actually had dropped 10%, from 8.8 to 7.9 per 100,000. The number of deaths had increased because the population had increased 41% and the average age was higher. During that same time, the death rates for cervical cancer dropped by 69% and those for uterine fundal cancer dropped by 52%. In 1988, the number of deaths from cervical cancer was 4443; the number of deaths from uterine fundal cancer was 5914.

The minimal reduction in the ovarian cancer death rate in the past 30 years means that we have to reevaluate our entire understanding of this disease with the hope of developing new approaches. With this aim, research goals have been proposed for academic departments of obstetrics and gynecology.[4] Unless there is an unexpected breakthrough in therapy, the only way to improve the prognosis of ovarian cancer is by early diagnosis when the cancer is still confined to the ovary. Prevention of ovarian cancer would be better yet.

The reason ovarian cancer is not diagnosed until the disease is advanced is that there are no signs of early disease or symptoms of early cancer. The most common early sign is abdominal enlargement due to ascites. In women over 40, unexplained vague digestive disturbances such as gas, discomfort, and distension may be due to ovarian cancer. There is usually no pain or abnormal bleeding.

Unfortunately, standard statistics cannot show recent changes in the incidence or mortality of ovarian cancer. This is not generally appreciated. There is no national cancer registry, and therefore the exact number of new cases of ovarian cancer is unknown. At different times there have been different methods for estimating the incidence. In 1973 the National Cancer Institute started the Surveillance, Epidemiology and End Results (SEER) program, which covered 10% of the U.S. population. Starting in 1979, estimates have been based on SEER incidence rates that are several years old, and these estimates are applied to current population estimates. The incidence estimate for 1992 was based on age-specific incidence rates from SEER 1986–1988 applied to the 1992 census population projections. Nevertheless, incidence rates can be compared from 1973 through 1988 from the SEER program.

Mortality estimates for 1992 are based on mortality data from 1982 through 1988 and were supplied by the Division of Vital Statistics, National Center for Health Statistics, Department of Health and Human Services.[2] Starting in 1981, the age-adjusted mortality per 100,000 was standardized to the 1970 census population distribution, instead of to the 1940 census.

Personal speculation is that if cancer mortality data is like maternal mortality data, there may be a 10 to 40% underreporting, in part due to late deaths and deaths from complications. In addition, since the mortality projection made at the beginning of 1992 by the American Cancer Society is based on the mortality rate no later than 1988, recent changes in mortality will not be evident. Correspondingly, any significant recent changes in cancer incidence will not be apparent.

Five-year relative survival rates published by the American Cancer Society in 1992 in fact are based on cases diagnosed during 1981–1987. Thus, recent therapeutic advances may not be evident.

This atlas is designed to serve as a reference for pathologists and as a bridge for communication with gynecologists and clinicians to improve patient care; it may also be a basic launching point for multidiscipline

investigations. The atlas has already stimulated some provocative questions, some examples of which follow.

The foundation of a study of a malignant disease is a study of its pathology. One of the problems in screening for ovarian carcinoma is how to consider the cystadenoma. "There is no evidence that cystadenoma represents a precursor lesion for invasive carcinoma."[3B] Purists believe that since the cystadenoma is not cancer, it should not be considered a positive finding. Others consider it to be potentially malignant and worthwhile discovering and removing. The interesting question is, does cancer start as cancer or does it develop from a preexisting lesion?

It has been assumed that the postmenopausal ovary is always small and quiescent. Ultrasonography has revealed a higher-than-expected incidence of unilocular ovarian cysts. What is the nature of these cysts? Are they neoplastic? Since they may recede, is there a functional endocrine activity that has not been recognized?

The apparent relatively rapid and asymptomatic spread and the poor prognosis of advanced ovarian cancer might be a clue to something else happening in addition to the general concept of ease of peritoneal spread. Is it possible that there is another factor relating to resistance to cancer spread that is expressed through the peritoneum? Could this unknown factor keep the cancer contained in the ovary and destroy shedding cancer cells? And could it be part of the reason for the good prognosis when early ovarian cancer is removed? Is it possible that some cases of early cancer remain confined to the ovary for long periods of time before discovery? Is the good result of early cancer surgery in part coincidental? Correspondingly, when this unknown factor is deficient, might it permit rapid discharge of cancer cells from the ovary and receptive growth on the peritoneum and in lymph nodes? (There might even be an analogy to endometriosis.) Therefore, normal peritoneum and normal areas of ovary in carcinoma patients might be worthwhile tissues for investigative pathology. Aside from the hospitality to shed cancer cells, how often does it happen that the peritoneum produces its own primary cancer with ovarian histology (which is suggested by advanced disease with only a small ovarian tumor)?

Is it possible that the early cancer has the initial genetic aberration of an exact uniform clone and is relatively less aggressive, while later, after further gene distortion and aneuploidy, it becomes more aggressive? Perhaps some subsequent cell variations start to produce lytic enzymes that facilitate spread. Does the early localized cancer have a different biology from the later advanced cancer?

A study of prognosis in stage III epithelial ovarian cancer utilizing the new 1988 International Federation of Gynecology and Obstetrics staging system was recently published.[5] Stage III is now subdivided into three substages by the volume of disease discovered at initial laparotomy: (a) tumor grossly limited to the true pelvis and negative nodes and microscopic seeding of abdominal peritoneal surfaces; (b) like substage a but with abdominal peritoneal implants less than 2 cm; and (c) abdominal implants larger than 2 cm and/or positive retroperitoneal or inguinal nodes. In this study, the mean age at diagnosis for stage IIIa was 40.5 years, for stage IIIb 51 years, and for stage IIIc 62 years! This remarkable decade between substages was not appreciated previously. "The age differential by substages suggests that the natural history of stage III disease is progressive over several decades."[5] This astonishing finding in a reputable journal has to be confirmed by others. It is not that ovarian cancer is simply more aggressive in older women, because even when corrected for age, the earlier subdivisions still have a better survival. The conclusion is extraordinary and different from conventional wisdom that assumes a uniformly rapidly growing and spreading tumor. It reinforces personal speculation that we do not know how long the tumor has existed before discovery, and that unknown biologic factors may play a role. Is it possible that sometimes the earlier tumor is less virulent, slower-growing, and different from the advanced tumor? Another unconventional suggestion of the report is that aggressive surgical debulking and bowel resection in advanced disease do not improve survival over biopsy alone! The authors realize that "a better understanding of the pathogenesis and molecular biology of ovarian cancer will be needed . . . ."[5]

The recognition of familial cancer syndromes and the gradual realization that it may not be very rare should alert the clinician to inquire about and examine other family members for ovarian cancer. It should also encourage examination of the patient and her family for associated cancers such as breast cancer (breast-ovarian syndrome) and cancer of the breast, colon, endometrium, etc. (Lynch II syndrome). This may supply the pathologist with biopsies of tissues that might have a malignant potential. With familial ovarian cancer, there may be as much as a 50% chance of ovarian cancer. This implies a genetic abnormality and a mechanism for activation. When such ovaries are removed prophylactically, they merit innovative oncogene pathology research. In addition, since primary peritoneal cancer with a histologic appearance similar to that of ovarian cancer may also occur, the peritoneum should also be studied in such families.

Despite the persistent dismal outlook in ovarian cancer, there has been a sudden and dramatic increase in exciting new concepts and research technologies. These include familial ovarian cancer; cancer as a gene disturbance; molecular biology; the origin of ovarian cancer; prophylactic oophorectomy; counseling; the role of laparoscopy; primary peritoneal ovarian cancer; attempts at early diagnosis; new chemotherapies; and questioning of the conventional assumptions of the value of very aggressive debulking and second-look laparotomy. This explosion in knowledge will translate into definite improvement in clinical results within the next decade. We hope that this atlas, aside from filling a conventional need, will also serve as a framework and launching platform for communication, investigation, and understanding.

The research pathologist and laboratory may be faced with a crisis in the future regarding confidentiality of individual results. As technology progresses with study of linkage, chromosomes, and oncogenes, familial ovarian cancer diagnosis will become generally available, as part of the overall increased knowledge of the genome. Will knowledge of predisposition to cancer affect a person's emotional stability, ability to obtain insurance, and major goals—higher education, employment, advancement, marriage, and having children?

## EPIDEMIOLOGY[6]

The risk of ovarian cancer increases with age, with the highest rates over age 60. There is a twofold increased risk in women who have never had children or who have had a previous breast cancer. Industrialized countries (except for Japan) have increased rates. Certain rare genetic conditions increase the risk. The risk is decreased with the use of oral contraceptives (OCs) and possibly with early age of first pregnancy and early menopause.

There are high rates of ovarian cancer in industrialized North America and Europe and low rates in developing countries and Japan. Worldwide, almost half of the 140,000 cases are in developing countries. In recent decades, the incidence and mortality have risen in low-risk areas. Late menopause might increase risk. Japanese women who move to the United States have the same increased ovarian cancer rate as other Americans after one or two generations.

The increased risk of ovarian cancer in women born since the late 1800s in developed countries might be due to industrialization itself or to decreased fertility and barrier contraception. Recent decreasing risk in developed countries may be related to OCs and coincidental oophorectomy in the older woman.

Over 60% of all primary ovarian neoplasms are common epithelial, about 20 to 25% are germ cell, and about 9% are sex cord–stromal tumors. About 90% of all ovarian cancers are common epithelial, in particular the serous endometrioid and mucinous adenocarcinoma. Because of this, the statistics of ovarian carcinoma are the statistics of common epithelial adenocarcinoma.

The annual incidence of ovarian cancer in the United States is 12 to 13 per 100,000 population, being slightly higher in whites than in blacks. Below age 45, blacks have a higher rate because they have more nonepithelial tumors.

Ovarian cancer incidence increases with age slowly and is unusual below age 40, in which case the rate is about 16 per 100,000. It then begins a steep rise to reach a peak of about 55 per 100,000 at age 70, and then levels because of oophorectomy. The median age of diagnosis is about 61, and the mean about 60.

The incidence of sex cord tumors parallel that of epithelial tumors but is at a much lower level.

Germ cell tumors are most common in the 20- to 24-year group, then markedly decline by about age 40, and thereafter have a slight rise.[7]

Among women who have had a laparotomy for ovarian neoplasm, the chance of malignancy is 13% in premenopausal women but 45% in postmenopausal women. There is a 12-fold increase in malignancy from ages 20 to 29 and from 60 to 69.[8]

Pregnancy definitely reduces the incidence of ovarian cancer; women have a relative risk of about 0.6 to 0.8 with one pregnancy, and with each additional pregnancy have about a 10% reduced risk.[7,9] Lactation tends to reduce the risk.

Involuntary infertility related to endocrine disturbance and persistent high gonadotropin levels or abnormal ovulation seems to be associated wtih increased ovarian cancer risk.[7,9]

Recently, three cases of ovarian serous adenocarcinoma of low malignant potential in infertile woman under 35 who had induction of ovulation with menotropin gonadotropin were reported.[10] The authors cited a previous report of seven cases of carcinoma following ovulation induction with clomiphene, which also increased gonadotropin levels. They questioned whether there is a link between infertility, ovulation induction, and ovarian carcinoma, or whether the increased surveillance resulted in earlier diagnosis.

It may be that the link was simply the previously suggested association of infertility with ovarian carcinoma. In general, carcinogens take a long time to act. It is possible that if there is an association, ovulation induction might cause a blossoming of a process under way. The young age of the patients might be accounted for if there were familial ovarian cancer; however, the family pedigree was not indicated in the report.

A recent large statistical study of 2197 white ovarian cancer patients in the United States indicated a decreasing risk with increasing numbers of pregnancies regardless of outcome, with increasing time of breast feeding, and with the use of OCs.[11] It suggests that these "induce biological changes that protect against ovarian malignancy." Tubal ligation sterilization and hysterectomy with the ovaries remaining reduced the risk. There was no change in risk with age at menarche, age at menopause, or the length of estrogen replacement therapy. There was an increased risk with the use of fertility drugs and in women who were never pregnant who had a long duration of sexual activity without contraception. It was suggested that "at most, a small fraction of the excess ovarian cancer risk among nulliparous women is due to infertility, and that any increased risk associated with infertility may be due to the use of fertility drugs."[11]

A statistical study of 327 white U.S. women with epithelial tumors of low malignant potential (LMP) showed a similar risk pattern for invasive cancer except for two differences.[12] The risk of LMP was "less clearly reduced among women who had used oral contraceptives and more clearly elevated among women with a history of infertility." The author noted that the former might be related to better screening that discovered the LMP tumors or to the use of low-dose OCs that might be less protective than older high-dose OCs and the latter might be due to fertility drugs or the type of infertility.

There have been two main theories regarding the pathogenesis of ovarian cancer.[13] One hypothesis is that an unknown sequela of ovulation ("incessant ovulation") increases the incidence of ovarian cancer and that pregnancy and OCs stop ovulation. The other hypothesis is that circulating gonadotropins (such circulation occurs in menopause) increase the incidence of ovarian cancer. Conflicting evidence includes the differential risk reduction of pregnancy versus OC use, the failure of postmenopausal estrogen replacement therapy to reduce the risk, and the slight if any risk change in relation to the ages of menarche and menopause.[13]

Hysterectomy with unilateral ovarian preservation reduces the risk of subsequent ovarian cancer by about half.[13] Some studies show that after 20 years the beneficial results disappear. The various theories to explain this disappearance include prophylactic removal of suspicious ovaries, alteration of ovarian blood flow, and prevention of the ascent of carcinogens from the vagina or perineum.[14] Talcum powder has been found in normal ovaries and ovarian tumors. In former years talc was contaminated with asbestos. Tubal ligation presumably would share the same putative protective mechanism.[7,9]

A literature review of OC use and the risk of ovarian

cancer indicated a relative risk of 0.64 with ever-use of OC, and therefore a 36% reduction in ovarian cancer risk.[15] The survey found a 10 to 12% decrease in risk with 1 year of OC use and a 50% decrease after 5 years of use. This benefit was in both nulliparous and parous women and lasted for at least 10 years after stopping the use of OCs. Although based on formerly used high-dose OCs, the decreased risk may also occur with the present low-dose OCs. The authors indicate that "the protective effect of OC against ovarian cancer risk should be considered in a woman's decision to use OC." Since the protection of parity is not modifiable, "only OC use offers an opportunity for primary prevention."[15] This paper raises the question of using OCs to prevent ovarian cancer. Neither hormone replacement therapy in menopause nor injected progestin contraceptive has any effect on ovarian cancer.[7]

There have been unverified suggestions that lactose deficiency and/or high yogurt consumption is associated with increase risk either as a marker or as a factor causing increased gonadotropin levels.[7]

Recent investigation suggests that epithelial ovarian cancer may be in part gonadotropin-dependent since it may have luteinizing hormone (LH) and follicle-stimulating hormone (FSH) receptors.[16] Gonadotropin-releasing hormone (GnRH) agonist therapy may be clinically helpful. There are also GnRH binding sites in ovarian cancer that might act as an autocrine regulator of ovarian cancer proliferation.[16]

There has been a suggestion that maternal exogenous hormone ingestion may increase the chance of germ cell cancers in the daughter.[7] A low level of serum $\alpha$-L-fucosidase may be a risk marker.

## GENETIC AND MOLECULAR ASPECTS OF OVARIAN CANCER

Prior to 1971, there were only scattered reports of rare families with a predisposition to ovarian cancer. Since then, there has been an explosive increase of reports of families with ovarian cancer, and a parallel increase in the study of involved genes and genetic factors.[9] Previously, it was thought that genetic ovarian cancer constituted only about 1% of ovarian cancer cases, the rest being sporadic. Although the vast majority are still considered sporadic, in December 1991, respected authorities wrote, "Although only 5–10% of all cases of ovarian cancer are attributed to hereditary causes, the greatest risk factor for ovarian cancer in any individual is a positive family history."[17]

Thus in 20 years there has been a 5- to 10-fold increase in the estimated prevalence of familial ovarian cancer. Some have echoed that "familial ovarian cancer is not a rare occurrence—as originally conceived from 1930 to 1970."[9] In addition, ovarian cancers are found to have abnormal genes and chromosomes both in tumor and in normal tissues. Therefore, even the sporadic cancers have abnormal genetic factors.

This is an extraordinary change in concept from a disease with a completely unknown etiology to a disease in which genetic factors are intimately involved.

Up to the present, even from large medical centers, interesting case reports of ovarian cancer, while indicating an unusual young age, have failed to give a pedigree.[10] This indicates that family history has been neglected.

With increased awareness of familial ovarian cancer, there will be more care in obtaining a family history. In all probability, this will increase the estimated prevalence of familial cancer.

Getting a reliable family history is difficult.[18] Ideally, three or four generations should be studied, with verification of ovarian cancer. This requires a large number of children, a population that does not move, and good record keeping. Unfortunately, the modern family is small and mobile and does not keep records.

It is essential to know the background incidence of cancer of the well general population.

With familial cancer, there is a tendency toward early age of onset, increased bilaterality, multifocal sites, multiple primary cancers, and poor prognosis.[19] There is autosomal dominance, and the abnormal genes may have paternal as well as maternal transmission.[19]

Inherited ovarian cancers occur 10 to 15 years earlier than sporadic, noninherited cancer. In the Gilda Radner Familial Ovarian Cancer Registry, the mean and median ages of mothers with cancer was 60.3 and 59.0, while the daughters with cancer were 47.5 and 47.7.[9] Such data may give clues as to the timing of genetic changes of ovarian somatic genes of the mother and germ cell genes of the daughter. They also suggest that at least some cases of sporadic cancer (mother) involve genetic abnormality.

Familial ovarian cancer tends to occur at younger ages (10 to 15 years) in following generations.[20] In six families with three-generation cancer, the median age of diagnosis of the grandmother was 68, of the mother 53.3, and of the daughter 45.

Lynch believes that in a hereditary ovarian cancer family, a woman with a first-degree relative in direct lineage (mother, daughter), with cancer has a 30 to 50% chance of cancer with an early-onset age of 45.[21] With a single first-degree relative with ovarian cancer, he finds that a woman has a relative risk of 3.6. With only a second-degree relative with ovarian cancer, he finds a relative risk of 2.9. According to Lynch's calculations, if the lifetime risk for the general population is 1.3%, having a first-degree relative with ovarian cancer gives a woman an ovarian cancer risk of 5%.

Piver and Recio indicate that with two or more first-degree relatives (mother, daughter, sister) with ovarian cancer, sisters and daughters may theoretically have as high as a 50% chance of developing ovarian cancer, because there seems to be an autosomal dominant pattern; however, because of variable penetrance, the actual lifetime risk might be about 40%.[20] This can be contrasted with the authors' estimate of a general population lifetime risk of 1.4%, or 1 in 70. With one first-degree relative with ovarian cancer, they found a risk of 4.5% and with one second-degree relative (grandmother, aunt) with ovarian cancer, a risk of 2.9%. For the following factors, the authors found a 2% risk: nulliparity, perineal talc exposure, infertility, high-fat diet, and previous breast cancer.

Others indicate that if the mother and daughter of a woman have ovarian cancer, the woman's risk is 100%.[19] If the mother and sister of a woman have ovarian cancer, they find that the woman's risk is 50%. If one first-degree and one second-degree relative have ovarian cancer, they find a risk of 25%; with only one first-degree relative with ovarian cancer, a risk of 10%; and with only one second-degree relative with ovarian cancer, a risk that may only be that of the general population. With relatives whose cancer developed before age 55, these authors find that a woman's risk is increased.

In familial ovarian cancer, there are three (or more) genotypes that predispose to ovarian cancer. The generally recognized three are[22]

1. Site-specific ovarian cancer
2. Ovarian cancer associated with breast cancer (breast-ovarian cancer syndrome)
3. Lynch Cancer Family Syndrome II (colon, endometrium, ovary, breast, stomach, urinary tract)

With familial ovarian-breast cancer, after the patient develops cancer in one site, there is an increased chance of developing cancer in the other site.[19] After breast cancer develops, there is an increased risk of a second primary cancer in the colon, endometrium, or ovary.

At present, family ovarian cancer diagnosis is based on family pedigree.[17,18] A genetic counselor may be helpful in defining the history since neglect of paternal history may confuse a site-specific ovarian cancer syndrome with a Cancer Family Syndrome (Lynch II).[17] In addition, pedigrees may be difficult to interpret.

Finally, there are the general population baseline lifetime risks of ovarian (about 1 to 2%), breast (11%), endometrial (8%), and colon cancer (5%).[19]

In an editorial on genetic risk in ovarian cancer, Lynch points out that one or more genes on chromosome 17 underlie a substantial proportion, but not all, of hereditary breast and ovarian cancer (HBOC) syndrome families.[21] The presence of these genes can be identified by linked polymorphic markers on multiple informative relatives of the HBOC family. Therefore, one may be more specific in identifying hereditary cancer families rather than relying on pedigree alone. Thus, the future may already be at hand, even though such testing is not yet generally available.

In one large kindred with familial breast-ovarian cancer syndrome, there was a high association with hereditary epidermolytic palmoplantar keratoderma (yellowish uniform hyperkeratosis surrounded by a red border of the entire palm and sole).[23]

It is possible that there may be a decrease in levels of serum $\alpha$-L-fucosidase, which may be a marker in patients with familial ovarian cancer.[19]

Based on family history, those at increased risk for ovarian cancer might be considered for counseling, screening to detect early disease, and prophylactic oophorectomy.

A reevaluation of three previous studies from the National Institutes of Health (NIH) indicated that women with one first-degree relative affected by ovarian cancer have an increased risk for such cancer, but at an age similar to that of the general population.[24] According to this analysis, women with several affected relatives have an increased risk of early-onset ovarian cancer. The authors found that about 20% of women from high-risk families had an onset younger than age 40, and the median age of onset was 47. Familial epithelial ovarian cancer is thought to be an autosomal dominant genetic defect with reduced penetrance. According to this reanalysis, high-risk factors for familial epithelial ovarian cancer include (1) two first-degree relatives; (2) an affected mother and an affected maternal second-degree relative; (3) an affected sister or daughter and any second-degree relative; and (4) many relatives with ovarian or breast cancer. For the above high-risk pedigree groups, those authors recommend prophylactic oophorectomy after the patient completes childbearing and/or by age 35. With only one first-degree relative with ovarian cancer, their estimate of risk to age 50 is about 0.5%, insufficient for current oophorectomy. After 50, the risk was found to be "substantially higher," but even then the authors were uncertain of the risk for familial ovarian epithelial cancer. It was difficult to make recommendations when considering families with multiple other tumors (breast, colon, endometrium). This study indicated that there is a 3.6 odds ratio for ovarian cancer in first-degree relatives with epithelial ovarian cancer. With premenopausal prophylactic oophorectomy, there may be an increased risk of cardiovascular disease and osteoporosis. In addition, despite oophorectomy, there may be a later primary peritoneal carcinomatosis with ovarian histology.

Recommended management for site-specific familial ovarian cancer includes genetic counseling at age 20, and screening by age 30 with ultrasound, physical pelvic examination, and serum Ca 125 testing every 6 months.[17] These authors recommend prophylactic oophorectomy after childbearing has been completed. Nevertheless, such surgery may still not prevent later peritoneal carcinomatosis.

When two or more first-degree relatives have ovarian cancer, Piver et al. advise prophylactic oophorectomy at age 35 if childbearing is completed.[9] Even though there is less risk with one first- and one second-degree or two second-degree relatives with ovarian cancer, they still recommend prophylactic oophorectomy.[20]

Lynch does not believe that prophylactic oophorectomy is appropriate if the only evidence is a single first- or second-degree relative with ovarian cancer.[21,22] He also recommends surveillance for breast, colon and endometrial cancer.

The Lynch Cancer Family Syndrome II involves multiple primary sites. Hereditary nonpolyposis colorectal cancer is the cause for about 5% of all colorectal cancer. It has two subdivisions: Lynch syndrome I, which is an autosomal dominant tendency to early-onset colorectal cancer, especially proximal to the splenic flexure; and Lynch syndrome II, which has in addition an excess of extracolonic cancer, particularly of the endometrium and ovary, and less often of the ureter, kidney, and stomach. Although, the colorectum is usually the first site of cancer, occasionally the first cancer may be of the endometrium or ovary. The diagnosis at present depends on a detailed family history including both maternal and paternal lineage.

All agree that even after prophylactic oophorectomy for familial ovarian cancer, there is a small risk of apparently primary peritoneal cystadenocarcinoma with a histologic appearance of ovarian cancer. Some estimate the risk to be 5%.[21,25]

These tumors have a different morphology from that of primary peritoneal mesothelioma.[26]

With prophylactic oophorectomy, a small focus of carcinoma and later peritoneal carcinomatosis,[17] borderline papillary ovarian carcinoma with endosalpingiosis of the peritoneum and pelvic lymph nodes,[27] and borderline ovarian carcinoma with node involvement with endosalpingeal-glandular inclusions may be discovered.[28] These patients tend to be young and infertile but often lack a pedigree history. The cases pose the question of peritoneal and node spread from a primary ovarian tumor versus simultaneous, independent, primary peritoneal or node malignant change.

Prophylactic oophorectomy may present an opportunity to investigate factors that might relate to oncogenesis, including protooncogenes and growth factors of the ovary and peritoneum.

In previous years, prophylactic oophorectomy required laparotomy. In recent years, advanced laparoscopy technique has made it feasible to do prophylactic oophorectomy. A frozen section should be available since there may already be an occult cancer present.

Thus we see extraordinary changes in clinical practice in recent years—the concept of familial ovarian cancer and the need for pedigree study (with the feasibility of more exact gene study at a later date), the concept of encouraging childbearing at an early age, the concept of prophylactic oophorectomy,[29] and the concept of laparoscopy for minimal invasive surgery.

Malignant transformation is associated with changes in genes and chromosomes, and this mechanism appears to be the "final common pathway."[30] Abnormalities may be inherited through germ cells and/or acquired through mutations of somatic ovarian surface cells. Malignant change requires the activation of several, rather than one, cancer-causing gene. "Epithelial ovarian cancer probably can occur due to activation of several different combinations of genes, such as *c-myc*, HER-2/*neu*, and p53, which may result in cancers that vary in their biologic and clinical characteristics."[30] Ovarian cancer cells have great variability in their chromosomes, including hypodiploidy; hyperdiploidy; breaks; deletions; translocations; loss of one gene allele (loss of heterozygosity), especially in chromosome 17; and gene amplification (increasing the number of genes).[19] Flow cytometric analysis of cellular DNA has made it possible to study DNA ploidy and the percentage of cells synthesizing DNA (S-phase fraction). High ploidy (aneuploid) and a large S-phase fraction are associated with worse prognosis.[31] Image analysis of neoplasm aneuploidy (DNA content) and abnormal nuclear texture (chromatin irregularity) correlate with prognosis in invasive and borderline ovarian tumors.[32] Cell flow cytometry of ascitic fluid for DNA aneuploidy in advanced papillary serous adenocarcinoma also had prognostic significance.[33] Early-onset dominant breast cancer is associated with the D17S74 locus on the long arm of chromosome 17q12-23. The cancer is presumably due to a mutation of the genes of that area. This same locus has now been associated with familial ovarian cancer as part of the familial breast-ovarian syndrome.[34] Amplification or overexpression of the HER-2/*neu* oncogene has been found in breast cancer and also in ovarian cancer. The greater the gene amplification, the worse the prognosis in ovarian cancer. The gene product may be a receptor for a growth factor.[17] It is located in the cell membrane. Prognosis problems in LMP cancers occur from nonspecific cytoplasmic staining and the inability to distinguish stage III cancer as a progression from stage I versus a simultaneous independent peritoneal carcinogenesis.[35]

Oncogenesis is a multistep sequence of mutations of dominantly acting protooncogenes (normally present genes that resemble retrovirus oncogenes) and mutations and reduction of functions of tumor-suppressing genes.[36] Most of these mutations are acquired rather than inherited. In ovarian cancer, there are extensive structural and numerical chromosomal changes proportional to neoplasm progression. Virulent ovarian cancers often have activation of the protooncogenes K-*ras*, *c-myc*, and *c*-erb B-2 (HER-2/*neu*). Cancers often show loss of putative tumor-suppressing genes for allele loci at chromosomes 11p, 17p, and 17q. Such losses often occur in other cancers also. An allelic loss on chromosome 6q may be specific to ovarian carcinoma. Familial breast-ovarian cancer may have a loss on chromosome 8q and of tumor-suppressing gene p53.[36]

Recent amazing molecular-genetic studies have shown that advanced ovarian epithelial cancer is a clonal disease developing from one mutant cell![37,38] Similar abnormal chromosomal karyotypes have been found in individual cases in bilateral ovarian cancers and omental implants. These tissues in individual cases all had the same p53 gene mutation[37] and the same patterns of allelic deletion of genes on chromosome 17.[38] Other evidence relates to the random inactivation of one X chromosome in each female somatic cell early in embryogenesis.[38] DNA probes of tissues in individual cases showed only paternal or maternal origin of the inactivated X chromosome rather than a mixture, thereby indicating a single-cell or unifocal origin. Cancers developing from different cells would have a 50:50 chance of having maternal or paternal patterns as is present in normal tissues.

It seems that an acquired genetic change gives an abnormal cell a growth advantage to form an original clone colony. "Subsequent changes in the genome of these cells may give rise to descendant cells which are more malignant, with further tumor progression."[37]

Molecular-genetic studies have not evaluated adequately early-stage and early-grade cancers, borderline cancers, and familial ovarian cancers. It is possible that the predispositions of the latter group might result in multifocal cancer origins with more than one clonal cell type.[37] This could explain apparent primary peritoneal cancers with ovarian serous histologic appearance.

## GENETIC ASPECTS OF NONEPITHELIAL OVARIAN TUMORS

The Peutz-Jeghers syndrome (autosomal dominant) of mucocutaneous pigmentation and intestinal hamartomas is associated with the ovarian sex cord tumor with annular tubules (SCTAT).[39,40] This neoplasm has features of both granulosa and Sertoli cell tumors. It is usually small and bilateral; however, there may be a malignant "adenoma malignum" of the cervix. Without the Peutz-Jeghers syndrome, the SCTAT tumors tend to be unilateral and large and may be malignant.

The basal cell nevus syndrome (also an autosomal dominant) has malignant epitheliomas developing at puberty, keratocytes of the jaw, and ovarian cysts and fibroadenomas.[19]

Ollier's disease (chondromatosis) and Maffucci's syndrome (enchondromatosis and hemangiomas) are associated with ovarian sex cord–stromal tumors (juvenile granulosa cell tumor, and Sertoli–Leydig cell tumors) in the first two decades of life.[41-44] This is part of a generalized mesodermal dysplasia. In later life, there is a more frequent sarcomatous change of enchondromas.

The phenotypic female androgen insensitivity (testicular feminization) patient with a short vagina and absent uterus and often with an inguinal hernia may have about a 20% chance of a gonadal cancer (usually seminoma) after age 30. Earlier, the chance is only about 5%. There may be a benign Sertoli cell adenoma.

Gynecologists usually recommend prophylactic gonadectomy after puberty. If, however, there is partial androgen insensitivity (incomplete syndrome) with an enlarged phallus, then gonadectomy is done before puberty to prevent puberty masculinization.

With 46, XY gonadol dysgenesis (Swyer syndrome), the patient is a phenotypic female who is tall, with primary amenorrhea, a small uterus, and streak ovaries.[45] There is no Turner's syndrome phenotype. There is a high incidence of gonadoblastoma and dysgerminoma. Swyer syndrome may be familial. The risk of malignant change increases with age and is about 10% at 15 years.

Even without the Y chromosome, rarely malignant ovarian change with 45, XO karyotype may occur in Turner's syndrome with Turner's phenotype.[46]

There are a new concept and a new standard of practice in managing dysgenetic gonads.[47] Previously, when both dysgenetic gonads were removed to prevent cancer, since childbirth was not possible it was customary to remove the uterus as well to avoid possible later endometrial cancer with estrogen replacement therapy. At present, the uterus is left in place because it is now possible with a donor egg, in-vitro fertilization, and hormonal preparation of the uterus for an agonadal woman to bear a child.

# THE EARLY DIAGNOSIS OF OVARIAN CANCER

Unfortunately, by and large, there is no early diagnosis of ovarian cancer. Nevertheless, rather than giving up in despair we must try to improve what we have been doing and explore new approaches at the same time.

Most ovarian tumors are found on physical examination. For most patients, the initial clinical visit is the basis of entrance into the medical care system.

There is no urgency in the early diagnosis of benign ovarian neoplasms. It is true that there may be torsion of a benign cyst that may cause ischemic necrosis of the involved ovary and tube creating an acute surgical emergency and the loss of these structures. There may be hemorrhage or other biologic accidents. Sometimes, huge growth of a benign cyst may destroy adjacent residual normal tissue and require oophorectomy rather than cystectomy. Hormone-producing tumors may cause precocious puberty, postmenopausal bleeding, or virilization. Eventually, large tumors may cause abdominal distension and pressure symptoms.

There is urgency in the early diagnosis of ovarian cancer before it spreads. Unfortunately, there are no early symptoms or signs of ovarian cancer when there is only slight enlargement of the ovary. Rarely, there are clues from hormonal activity or biologic accidents. Previously, it was assumed that the postmenopausal ovary was quiescent and that the "palpable ovarian syndrome" (ovary of premenopausal size rather than the usual nonpalpable atrophic ovary) was an indication for surgical exploration. It is now recognized that the postmenopausal ovary may have benign functional nonneoplastic cysts, and most enlargements less than 5 cm are not malignant. This, of course, raises important questions about the biology and anatomy of the normal postmenopausal ovary and about our past assumptions.

When symptoms occur in ovarian cancer, the disease is already advanced. There may be debilitation; pain; anorexia; vomiting; weight loss; abdominal distension; pressure; malnutrition; thin arms and legs; lymphatic obstruction causing edematous legs; abnormal vaginal bleeding; fever; and back pain. Earlier milder preceding symptoms are vague, with abdominal discomfort, indigestion, nausea, and gastrointestinal discomfort. Barber emphasizes dyspepsia, loss of appetite, indigestion, gas, distension, history of ovarian dysfunction, and age over 40.[48] Most such mild symptoms in the general population are functional and suggest gallbladder, stomach, or intestinal causes. Sometimes with ovarian cancer, there may be a worsening of a hiatus hernia, probably due to mild ascites. There may be vaginal abnormal, irregular or heavy, bleeding (premenopausal and also postmenopausal bleeding). Torsion, bleeding, and wall penetration may occur in the tumor.

"Routine pelvic examinations detect only 1 ovarian cancer in 10,000 asymptomatic women."[49] Obviously, to organize pelvic examination as a screening technique for ovarian cancer is not feasible. "However, pelvic examination remains the most practical means of detecting early disease."[49] Pelvic examination should be part of a general, often annual, physical examination. If pelvic examination is used as a screening test for high-risk cases, then perhaps it should be done at 4- to 6-month intervals.

In taking the history notice is made of age, onset menarche, menstrual record, menopause, parity, use of OCs, previous abdominal surgery, previous breast surgery, and any vague abdominal disturbance. A careful family history is obtained for malignancy, especially ovarian, breast, colon, and uterine, but also for cancer in male members.

Recommendation is made for routine mammography and colonoscopy or sigmoidoscopy depending on usual criteria. Breast self-examination is taught for monthly examinations after menstruation.

On physical examination of patients with ovarian cancer, 1 to 2% of patients have a negative examination, 20 to 30% are found to have clinical ascites, and 40 to 75% are found to have a palpable abdominal mass.[50A] There may be a pleural effusion and distant metastases to the skin or lymph nodes (inguinal, supraclavicular, or axillary). Abdominal palpation may show "omental cake" masses of carcinomatous metastases or periumbilical metastases. Distension may also be found to be due to partial bowel obstruction. These findings apply to the usual situation of discovery of the ovarian cancer at an advanced stage. Depending on the stage, difficulty of examination, and experience of the examiner, the chance of missing an ovarian cancer on examination has been estimated from $1/3$ to $2/3$. "The most common mistaken preoperative diagnosis is uterine fibroids,"[5B] which may happen in about 2.5% of "fibroid" cases.

Ascites may cause abdominal distension, a fluid wave, and shifting dullness. Infrequently, a happy discovery is Meigs's syndrome of an ovarian fibroma with ascites and pleural fluid; congenital hepatic cysts simulating metastases on liver scanning (personal case); or a sigmoid-ovarian abscess due to diverticulitis or a perforating chicken bone simulating ovarian cancer (personal case).

Physical examination is the traditional mainstay of the physician, yet it has not led to earlier diagnosis or improved the survival rate of ovarian cancer. Almost all ultrasound screening reports have included ovarian carcinomas that were not palpated.

Slight enlargement of the ovary is asymptomatic and may be difficult or impossible to palpate, but it can usually be detected by ultrasound. Ultrasound has a sensitivity of 83%, while physical examination has a sensitivity of 67%.[51] Both have a similar specificity of about 95%.

Among normal postmenopausal women, 87% of ovaries could be identified by ultrasound, but only in 30% could the ovaries be palpated on physical examination.[52] "Even under optimal circumstances, the patient with symptomatic ovarian cancer may have a negative pelvic examination."[50B]

Nevertheless, even if not ideal, physical examination should not be discarded, and every effort should be made to improve its sensitivity in detecting ovarian enlargement.

The American Cancer Society recently did a disservice in recommending cervical cytology testing at 3-year intervals after three prior normal cytology reports. This was based on a statistical analysis assuming that the cytology smear would be made properly and interpreted by experts. Unfortunately, the assumption was incorrect. It was also incorrect in not considering the epidemic of papilloma viruses that cause flat condyloma of the cervix and atypia, and probably are involved with malignant transformation. The problem as it relates to ovarian cancer is that the average woman, and sometimes the general physician, might erroneously conclude that a pelvic examination is only needed at 3-year intervals.

Physical pelvic examinations should be done at least once a year and more often in increased-risk groups.

Another issue is the quality of the pelvic examination. Most physicians were never taught how to do a pelvic examination correctly. They cannot be expected to palpate small enlargements that a gynecologist should be able to find.

The teaching of history taking and physical examination is looked down upon by many, especially since it has not changed very much over the decades. It is part of the malady of giving only lip service to teaching, while basing promotions on publications. The development of modern imaging techniques has also reduced the stature of the physical examination. Advances in physiology and molecular biology are the glamorous aspects of medicine today and capture our interests. Nevertheless, history taking and physical examination are still the keystones of abdominal and pelvic diagnosis. They are the first steps by which patients enter the medical system and are triaged into routine checkups, more careful observation, or immediate testing. This is

the essence of cost-effective care based on a careful clinical evaluation by the individual physician.

All physicians who care for women should learn how to do good physical pelvic examinations. Although simple, some concepts are worth repeating. The patient should have an empty bladder and bowel. There is nothing wrong with having the patient return after an enema if stool prevents an adequate examination. The patient should be relaxed and not have the tense abdominal wall of anxiety and fear.

The gynecologic examination begins after a history and general physical examination. The gynecologic examination includes the breast. The abdomen is inspected, palpated gently and then more vigorously, percussed, and, if appropriate, tested for shifting dullness and fluid wave. Whereas textbooks show pictures of two fingers in the vagina, for the narrow vagina, one finger is used. The vaginal fingers are for sensing—not for pushing and provoking pain and spasm of the abdominal wall. To emphasize this some instructors indicate that the elbow of the examiner should rest on the knee of the examiner to ensure that the examining arm merely rested (the examiner's foot was on the step of the table). The opposite hand palpated the abdomen and gently pushed down the uterus and adnexa into the pelvis, making contact with the vaginal examination fingers. The cervix and uterus were then identified and the remainder was therefore adnexal. In general, uterine leiomyomas are rigidly fixed to the uterus and move with it while ovarian masses do not.

Unfortunately, many gynecologists do not do routine rectovaginal bimanual examinations with the second (index) finger in the vagina, the third (large) finger in the rectum, and the opposite hand on the abdomen. They may not have been trained to do this routinely, and they do not wish to cause discomfort to the patient. Nevertheless, this examination should be done, especially when the patient is seen infrequently. The rectal examination also affords an opportunity to do a stool test for occult blood. Any nodularity of the cul-de-sac pouch of Douglas, the sacrouterine ligaments, the rectovaginal septum, the posterior wall of the uterus, and the parametria should be noticed. Benign ovarian tumors tend to be smooth, cystic, mobile, unilateral, and less than 5 cm. Malignant tumors tend to be solid, irregular, larger, and bilateral, but there is great variation. No longer allowed to grow, in former years massive abdominal enlargement was due to unilateral, benign ovarian mucinous cystadenoma. This can give a fluid wave, as does myxoma peritonei.

Ideally, the same physician-gynecologist should do repeat examinations, whether for routine follow-up or for further evaluation. A good method of improving physical examination skills (although not generally available) is to examine patients preoperatively and again while the patients are under anesthesia, and finally to be present at the laparatomy or laparoscopy.

Should there be concern, the physician has to decide on further testing and repeat examination. The usual imaging requested is abdominal-pelvic sonography and, more recently, transvaginal sonography. Sonography is readily available, convenient, noninvasive and without radiation exposure, and it can be repeated without limitations. The only problem is the cost. The physician always faces the threat of legal action for negligence for failure of early diagnosis. It may be that the federal government and insurance companies may eventually dictate cost-effectiveness utilization of screening tests as part of "managed medical care." This may make the physical examination more critical—is the ultrasound ordered as a screening test or is it ordered because there is a palpable pelvic-abdominal mass or symptoms? Transvaginal color-directed Doppler flow measurements are more expensive than simple morphologic imaging; however, such a cost is more readily acceptable if an ovarian tumor has already been discovered and there is a question of whether it is malignant.

High-risk family history cases require more careful surveillance than routine cases.

Most discovered adnexal masses are not ovarian cancer. The usual investigation includes transvaginal ultrasound, if possible with Doppler color flow. About 10% of ovarian carcinoma is metastatic, often from the colon or breast.

## SCREENING FOR OVARIAN CANCER

Despite the lack of a standard screening procedure, who should be screened? The highest risk would be the ovarian cancer families, in which the risk may be as high as 50%.

There is a large group in which there is a family history of cancer but in which because of a lack of history, small size of family, or lack of agreement on the definition of a family cancer syndrome there is no family cancer syndrome diagnosis. An example is the woman who knows of one first-degree relative with ovarian cancer, which of itself confers a 5% risk. There may be a spectrum of family involvement and therefore a spectrum of risk. There may also be overlaps with possible breast-ovary familial cancer syndrome or familial cancer Lynch II (breast, colon, and uterus as well as ovary).

Another group with increased risk of ovarian cancer consists of women who have already had breast or colon carcinoma (if there was previous endometrial carci-

noma, the ovaries would probably already have been removed). It is possible that any extraovarian cancer may predispose to later new primary ovarian cancer. Furthermore, with any primary cancer elsewhere, there may be metastatic ovarian cancer.

Finally, there is the postmenopausal woman who was never pregnant, who never took contraceptive pills, who lives in an industrial society in northern Europe or North America.

There is a consensus that there is no satisfactory method to screen the asymptomatic general population for ovarian cancer. The high incidence of false-positive results "do not justify the use of Ca 125 or ultrasound for screening asymptomatic women for ovarian cancer, especially since the annual incidence of ovarian cancer for woman over age 45 in the United States is about 40 per 100,000."[52]

Until we have the results of a randomized, controlled study to determine the effect on mortality of serum screening for early-stage disease, "the efficacy of potential tests for ovarian cancer will remain unproven and they should not be used to screen apparently healthy women outside of research protocols."[53]

In spite of this pessimistic outlook, many workers (including the above) are actively searching for and improving screening techniques. Investigation has centered mainly on the Ca 125 blood test and ultrasound.

Proponents of screening, based on small numbers of reports and the assumption that finding ovarian cancer before it has spread beyond the ovary and treating it at that time will improve survival, suggest that diagnosis of early cancer should improve survival. Despite an unproven ability to reduce mortality by early discovery, screening by pelvic examination, Ca 125, and ultrasound is being urged on television by the Gilda Radner Ovarian Cancer Group.

Because ovarian cancer is not common and because of a lack of specificity, screening is expensive. Government and medical insurance groups will probably not consider present screening to be "cost-effective" in plans to reduce health care costs.

In standard clinical practice, routine screening of U.S women over the age of 45 years with serum Ca 125 and ultrasound is not recommended since it would cost about $14 billion. Each case of stage I ovarian cancer detected would cost almost $1 million. Therefore, ovarian cancer screening for the asymptomatic general population is done primarily for research.[3B] Nevertheless, it is possible that there might be unanticipated economic factors such as: widespread use of screening technology reducing the cost and the economic stimulus of widespread screening.

In the United Kingdom and the United States, the incidence of ovarian cancer in women aged 45 years or over is 40 per 100,000 per year.[3B] If there were an annual screening test with 100% sensitivity, it would require 99.6% specificity to have a positive predictive value of 10%. This means for each case of ovarian cancer there would be 9 false-positives. Most clinicians would consider this to be the absolute minimal reliability. Only 1 of 67 abnormal transabdominal ultrasound examinations is due to ovarian cancer.

In screening for ovarian cancer, the specificity of pelvic examination is 97.3%, that of abdominal ultrasound 94.6%, and that of Ca 125 97.0%. These are all relatively poor.

Various strategies are being studied to improve the specificity of Ca 125 screening by using serial testing, by combining it with other serum markers for initial screening, and by adding pelvic examination and ultrasound.[53]

If screening is done for the general population, most recommend it for postmenopausal women over 50 years, who have less functional change in ovarian volume on ultrasonography, who have less chance of a benign condition's elevating the serum Ca 125 level, and who have an increased prevalence of ovarian cancer. With familial ovarian cancer, screening may be started about age 30.

Current investigation has centered on (1) molecular biology to attempt to prevent, diagnose early, and improve treatment of ovarian cancer, (2) clinical early detection by serum markers and ultrasonography, and (3) clinical differentiation of benign versus malignant ovarian masses, especially with ultrasound morphology, color flow, and Doppler waveform analysis.

It has been suggested that finding the genes involved in familial ovarian cancer might give "disease identification of cancer families and also women who are at high risk in the general population. Knowledge of the early biochemical events may eventually lead to the development of an immunochemical self-test for early ovarian oncogenesis."[54]

In evaluation ovarian cancer screening, some have evaluated only the bottom line—how many ovarian cancers were discovered.[3B] They feel that the discovery of benign neoplasms is almost inconsequential. They also feel that it has never been demonstrated that malignant neoplasms originate from benign neoplasms. On the other hand, to prevent complications (torsion, etc.) clinical gynecologists have always felt justified in removing ovarian neoplasms even knowing that they are benign and asymptomatic, unless the patient's general health prevents surgery.

Clinical gynecologists also recognize that rarely a benign dermoid may have a focus of squamous cell or other carcinoma. In addition, a large apparently benign ovarian serous cystadenoma at frozen section may later be found with further sectioning to have a malignant area. Thus the clinician has always had a feeling that benign neoplasms sometimes may become malignant. The study of Bourne et al. tends to confirm this feeling.[54]

Perhaps we have underestimated the incidence of primary or simultaneous serous peritoneal cystadenocarcinoma among cases of ovarian cancer. Perhaps this might explain a subgroup with apparent rapid spread, lack of symptoms from a primary large ovarian mass, and poor prognosis. Screening might detect such cases.

## Ca 125

Ca 125 is a high-molecular-weight cell surface glycoprotein complex of molecules that is present in forms varying from 220 to over 1000 kD.[55] Although, many other cell surface glycoproteins are mucins, it is not, because it has less than 50% carbohydrate. To date the Ca 125 gene has not been identified. There is no pure preparation of Ca 125.[55]

The Ca 125 antigen is identified by OC 125, a mouse monoclonal antibody, which was produced from a mouse spleen cell that was immunized by a human papillary ovarian cystadenocarcinoma cell line by Bast et al.[56]

The concentration of Ca 125 is expressed in arbitrary units per milliliter.[57] The upper normal is 35 U/ml. The serum half-life is about 4.5 days.

Although it was discovered by using an antibody to ovarian cancer, the Ca 125 antigen complex is normally found in cells derived from the coelomic epithelium—müllerian duct structures, fallopian tube, endometrium, decidua, endocervix, peritoneum, pleura, and pericardium as well as bronchus and amniotic epithelium.

The Ca 125 antigen may have an as-yet-undescribed physiologic role.[56] Although originally thought not to be present in normal ovarian surface epithelium, it may be present in some areas. It is also present to some extent in the epithelia of the pancreas, colon, gallbladder, stomach, lung, and kidney.

Elevated Ca 125 levels may occur in 6% of normal premenopausal women, 3.4% of perimenopausal women, and 3% of postmenopausal women.[57,58] Some indicate that there is an overall 1 to 3% chance that a normal woman will have an elevated level of Ca 125.[55]

About 1% of general obstetric-gynecologic cases without malignancy may have a Ca 125 level of over 65 U/ml.[8]

Ca 125 levels may be elevated with nonmalignant gynecologic conditions such as endometriosis, adenomyosis, leiomyoma, acute pelvic inflammatory disease, early pregnancy, menstruation, and benign ovarian cysts.

In the follicular phase the mean serum Ca 125 level of normal women was found to be 12.2 ± 4.1, while during menses it was 15.8 ± 7.3.[59] During menstruation with mild endometriosis, the Ca 125 level was 22.6 ± 12.4, with moderate endometriosis it was 33.8 ± 38.2, and with severe endometriosis it was 68.7 ± 43.0.

With benign ovarian stromal tumors without ascites, the Ca 125 level is normal.[60] With ascites the Ca 125 levels with ovarian stromal tumors (Meigs's syndrome) may be increased from 329 to 5000 U/ml.[60]

Elevated Ca 125 levels may occur in nonmalignant general medical conditions such as peritonitis, pancreatitis, cirrhosis of the liver and renal failure, and after laparotomy.[52,56]

Original studies did not find Ca 125 on ovarian surface epithelium, although it was present in ovarian surface epithelial cells lining inclusion cysts, papillary excrescences, and adhesions where metaplasia had occurred.[56] Recent investigation has shown that Ca 125, in fact, may occur in some normal ovarian epithelium.[56]

Since most ovarian cancers are serous and discovered in an advanced stage, the preoperative serum Ca 125 level is elevated in about 85% of cases.[56] However, in stage I cases in which the cancer is confined to the ovary, the level is elevated in only 50% of cases. In stage II the level is elevated 90%, stage III 92%, and stage IV 94%.

Therefore, the Ca 125 level is inherently not sufficiently sensitive to be an ovarian cancer screening test.

Ca 125 antigen is a tumor marker and like others is tumor-associated and not tumor-specific. Since Ca 125 was derived from serous carcinoma, it is understandable that it is expressed less with mucinous carcinoma.[56] About 69% of mucinous carcinoma patients have elevated Ca 125 levels. Interestingly, with endometrial ovarian carcinoma, the percentage with elevated Ca 125 levels is 75%, with clear cell carcinoma it is 78%, and with undifferentiated carcinoma it is 88%.

Ca 125 levels are often increased with other gynecologic cancers of the endometrium, fallopian tube, and endocervix.[56] Ca 125 levels may also be increased with cancers of the pancreas, colon, gallbladder, lung, breast, stomach, liver, and kidney.

Despite early hopes that the Ca 125 antigen could be used as a serum screening test for ovarian cancer, this test has not materialized. To be clinically acceptable, a screening test would have to have a minimum 10% positive predictive value.[53,56] This would require a 100% sensitivity and a 99.6% specificity for ovarian cancer, which in 45-year-old women has an incidence of 40 per 100,000 per year.

The specificity of a single serum Ca 125 elevation is only 97%.[56] This would result in 75 false-positives for each case of ovarian cancer. A single Ca 125 test does

not have sufficient sensitivity or specificity to be a suitable screening test. It may have a role in tests of several tumor markers, in serial testing, and in association with ultrasound.

The specificity of clinical pelvic examination alone is 97.3% and of abdominal ultrasound alone is 94.6%.[53] Combining Ca 125 testing with ultrasound produced a specificity of 99.6% and with pelvic examinations added reached 100% in one study.[56]

Unfortunately, "the sensitivity of serum Ca 125 measurement alone or in combination with other tests for preclinical early-stage ovarian cancer is unknown. However, it is unlikely to be higher than the figure of 53% established for clinically diagnosed stage I disease."[56]

There is retrospective data indicating that Ca 125 levels of women who later (1 to 143 months) developed ovarian cancer were greater than those in controls.[56] Individual cases may have had levels over 65 U/ml within 28 months of cancer diagnosis.

It is hoped that the specificity of screening of asymptomatic postmenopausal women for ovarian cancer with serum tumor-associated antigens can be increased to suitable levels by serial and/or combination measurements.[53] The specificity of Ca 125 at 30 U/ml and at 50 U/ml was increased from 97.0% and 99.5%, respectively, to 98.9% and 99.9% when either a Ca 15-3 level greater than 30 U/ml or a serum marker TAG 72.3 level greater than 10 U/ml was added. With Ca 125 alone, a level over 50 U/ml initially and over 30 U/ml at a 3-month follow-up gave a 99.6% specificity.[53] Levels of over 30 U/ml initially and over 30 U/ml at 3 months have a 98.9% specificity. In general, those without cancer with initially elevated levels tended to return to normal at follow-up. Those with cancer and an initially elevated level would be expected to have the levels rise.

While Ca 125 is the usual tumor marker for serous cystadenocarcinoma, the CA 72-4 (TAG 72) antigen may be useful with both mucinous and serous cystadenocarcinoma.[61] There may be about a 20% false-negative result with Ca 125, especially in mucinous tumors.[62]

Combinations of serum tumor markers have been tried to differentiate epithelial ovarian cancer from benign ovarian masses.

Using a cutoff of 65 U/ml instead of the usual 35 U/ml, the sensitivity decreased only slightly from 82.2 to 75.6%, while the specificity increased significantly from 67.3 to 86.6% and a diagnostic accuracy of 83.7% was obtained for epithelial ovarian cancer.[62] In patients over age 50, the combination of Ca 125 (with a 65 U/ml cutoff) and Ca 19.9 (antigen associated with colon carcinoma and especially mucinous ovarian cancer) testing increased the sensitivity from 81.1% to 93.2% and slightly lowered the specificity from 86.0% to

78.9%. In stages III and IV compared with stages I and II, the Ca 125 sensitivity with a 35 U/ml cutoff was 92.8% versus 19.0%, and with a 65 U/ml cutoff it was 71.2% versus 11.1%.

A new class of serum tumor markers, the highly glycosylated high-molecular-weight mucins, when combined with Ca 125, may increase the sensitivity and specificity of tests.[63]

There is continuing research in histologic monoclonal antibody keratin markers.

When ovarian surface epithelial (mesothelial) cells undergo metaplastic change to cystadenoma and carcinoma, they synthesize a 200-kD (non–Ca 125) glycoprotein recognized by a monoclonal antibody, produce ovarian carcinoma–associated antigens, and focally produce keratin 4 and/or 13.[64]

Preoperative Ca 125 levels in borderline ovarian tumors correlated with the extent of the cancer, with both serous and mucinous tumors.[65] With stage I, 25 to 40% of the patients had elevated Ca 125 levels; with spread beyond the ovary, 92 to 100% had elevated levels.

In general, peritoneal fluid Ca 125 levels are higher than serum levels in benign and malignant conditions. "One can speculate that metastases within the peritoneal cavity are the source of the antigen."[66] With cancer, when peritoneal fluid (ascites) Ca 125 levels were measured, there was 96% sensitivity and 99% specificity using values over 200 U/ml. With ascites, serum Ca 125 levels greater than 35 U/ml had a sensitivity of 99% and a specificity of 94%. Only 2 of 165 cases with benign conditions had peritoneal fluid levels over 200 U/ml. Only 2 of 35 cancer cases had ascitic fluid levels less than 200 U/ml. It is possible that peritoneal fluid Ca 125 levels may have value in management.

The normal cutoff level of peritoneal Ca 125 levels is 250 U/ml.[67] Cancer cases have higher levels, especially with bulky tumors. Survival is inversely related to peritoneal fluid levels.

Personal speculation is that the marked increase in serum levels of Ca 125 from stage I to stage II might be due not only to a larger tumor mass and metastatic morphology but also to peritoneal irritation. Ca 125 serum levels may be increased in peritonitis and pelvic inflammatory disease. Personal observation of advanced cancer shows a variation of nontumor areas of peritoneum from a bland, quiet appearance to an angry, reactive inflamed appearance.

Ca 125 levels may also be increased in Meigs's syndrome of ovarian fibroma and benign stromal tumors with ascites, but not with stromal tumors within ascites.[60] Thus it would be of interest to study noncancerous areas of peritoneum of ovarian cancer cases for ascites production, inflammatory reaction, receptivity to tumor implantation, and propensity for tumor formation.

What is the value of measuring levels of serum Ca 125? As an individual single screen for ovarian cancer, most feel that it should not be done. It may be helpful in management.

Ca 125 may have value in the postmenopausal woman who has already been found to have an enlarged ovarian mass.[55] A Ca 125 level of over 50 to 65 U/ml has an 80 to 90% chance of indicating an ovarian cancer. Therefore, a gynecologic oncologist should be available at the initial laparotomy for a staging and cytoreduction. Since the negative predictive value is only about 75%, the mass may still be malignant despite a normal Ca 125 level.

Serum Ca 125 levels may be helpful in management.[68] In general, the levels may correlate with tumor load in epithelial cancer. With a preoperative level less than 65 U/ml there may be a better prognosis.

Even with those cancer cases with preoperative levels below 65 U/ml, monitoring of serum Ca levels is useful in the early diagnosis of progressive disease.[69]

"The post-operative Ca 125 level is of independent prognostic significance."[88] A normal or slightly elevated level had a better prognosis.

Ca 125 levels before chemotherapy had no prognostic significance.[70] With high levels of Ca 125 (over 100 U/ml) one month after the third course of chemotherapy, the median survival was 7 months. If the Ca 125 level was 10 U/ml or less, there was a 50% 5-year survival; with an intermediate Ca 125 level, there was a median survival of 22 months. Increasing or maintained high levels are a poor prognostic sign and predictive of persistent disease, although a normal Ca 125 level does not guarantee no disease.[55] A progressively high Ca 125 level after remission indicates recurrence 3 months before other noninvasive methods are able to detect it. A rapid decrease in Ca 125 levels during therapy to normal levels is a favorable sign.

A recent development was the discovery that explains the falsely elevated Ca 125 level that is sometimes found in normal women.[71] The antigenic nature of Ca 125 in normal women is different from that in women with ovarian cancer. The false-elevation patients have normal levels of Ca 130, a different antigenic determinant on the same Ca 125 antigen molecule. With cancer there is an increase in both Ca 125 and Ca 130.

## ULTRASOUND

The major clinical advance in the diagnosis of ovarian tumors has been in ultrasonography. It is convenient, readily available, relatively inexpensive compared with computerized tomography, x-ray examination, or magnetic resonance imaging, and usually gives just as good or better imaging as the latter two modalities.

It has been used for

1. Screening for ovarian cancer in asymptomatic women.
2. Diagnostic testing for symptomatic women.
3. Imaging of ovarian masses already discovered to determine whether the mass is an ovarian neoplasm and whether it is benign or malignant.
4. Management of ovarian tumors with a suspicion of malignancy: the kidneys are checked for obstruction, the liver for metastases, the omentum for infiltration, and the peritoneal cavity for ascites. Preparation may be made for surgical peritoneal washings, frozen section, and the availability of a gynecologic oncologist. The most common ovarian neoplasm is the benign mature cystic teratoma or dermoid cyst, which can usually be diagnosed by ultrasound. Although there is a small chance of secondary malignant transformation, a lower abdominal transverse incision might be considered. A significant problem is the ovarian enlargement in the postmenopausal woman. Previously, it was assumed that all required laparotomy and removal. Increasing experience has shown that most are benign. One option is continued observation with serial sonography. Another option is laparoscopy with removal of the enlarged ovary without rupturing it, immediate frozen section, and possible immediate laparotomy for surgical staging. Ultrasound is also useful in monitoring therapy and recurrences.

The traditional ultrasound imaging used extensively in evaluating gynecologic conditions has been via the abdominal and lower abdominal, or pelvic, approach. It uses low-frequency transducers to reach the entire pelvis, resulting in a loss of image quality, especially in the obese woman. In addition, distended loops of bowel create artifacts and cast shadows. Finally, it requires time and patient discomfort for bladder filling to create a visual contrast.

About 1990, the transvaginal approach became popular. The transducer was closer to the ovarian tumor, and high-frequency ultrasound could be used because of shorter distance, with resulting improvement in image quality and definition. The problems of obesity and intestinal gas were reduced. With an empty bladder, the procedure is faster and with much less discomfort for the patient.[51] The disadvantage of transvaginal ultrasonography is the limitation of the field, and therefore, an ovarian tumor that is high or large may require additional abdominal-pelvic sonography to examine the up-

per part of the tumor. Additional abdominal-pelvic sonography would also be required to image the abdomen (kidneys, liver, omental metastases). Another disadvantage of the transvaginal approach, which has not been discussed in the literature, is the anxiety that some patients have when someone other than their gynecologist does a vaginal examination. Therefore, the patient should be alerted in advance. Transvaginal probing may not be possible with a stenotic vagina in a postmenopausal woman or a young girl. The ideal procedure for transvaginal sonography, which has not been discussed in the literature, is to have an experienced physician do the pelvic examination at the same time as manipulating the transducer. This reduces the chance of missing a small mass and gives some correlation between fixation, consistency, and tenderness. In some facilities, the sonography is done automatically by a technician, who simply empirically, without examination, takes several representative angle views with the transducer, and the films are later interpreted by a radiologist. This may reduce the reliability of such imaging, but the procedure may not be indicated in publications.

About 1991, the transvaginal approach was improved by the addition of color flow and Doppler waveform analysis. With ultrasound screening, it is important to keep the following definitions in mind:[72]

$$\text{Sensitivity} = \frac{\text{true positive}}{\text{true positive} + \text{false negative}}$$

$$\text{Specificity} = \frac{\text{true negative}}{\text{true negative} + \text{false positive}}$$

$$\text{Positive predictive value} = \frac{\text{true positive}}{\text{true positive} + \text{false positive}}$$

$$\text{Negative predictive value} = \frac{\text{true negative}}{\text{true negative} + \text{false negative}}$$

Traditional sonographic indications of malignancy include irregular solid areas, thick septae, poorly defined margins, matted loops of intestine, and ascites. The use of transabdominal ultrasound as a screening test for ovarian cancer was first proposed by Stuart Campbell and coworkers at King's College in London.[72,73] Among 5749 self-selected asymptomatic women, 10.1% had ovarian enlargement detected on three serial screens. With follow-up ultrasound, there was a reduction to 5.9%, with premenopausal reduction of cases with ovarian enlargement detected four times more frequent than postmenopausal reduction. Four women had metastatic ovarian cancer; three were found at screen 1, and one was found at screen 2. Five women (0.1%) had primary ovarian cancers, two at screen 1 and three at screen 2. Four were stage Ia and one was stage Ib. All the primary cancers were cured. The specificity was 97.7%, and the false-positive rate was 2.3%. The odds that a positive screening would indicate an ovarian tumor were 1:2, the odds for any ovarian cancer were 1:37, and for a primary ovarian cancer 1:67. These authors defined normal ovarian size in postmenopausal women. The normal ovary had a smooth ovoid outline and a uniform, low-level echogenicity. The ovarian volume was calculated as $\pi/6 \times$ maximum transverse diameter $\times$ antero-posterior $\times$ longitudinal. The scan was positive if any of the following three factors was abnormal: morphology (hyper or hypoechogenecity), irregular outline, or volume over 20 ml. The same group later commented that detection of early cancer should be either abnormal morphology or a volume more than 96th percentile at scan 1 followed by an increased volume at scan 2; or abnormal morphology at scan 1 followed by increase in volume at scan 2. The maximum ovarian volumn was analyzed according to age and menstrual status. "Any woman with a positive result at scan 1 should be rescanned as soon as possible after 20 days have elapsed."[74]

In a series of 805 women who attended an outpatient clinic, routine abdominal sonography showed abnormalities in 83.[75] Repeat scanning confirmed persistence in 50. There were 5 ovarian cystadenomas and one caecal cancer. There were 1 ovarian cancer and 2 borderline cancers, none of the three were clinically palpable.

It has been estimated that routine ultrasound screening of asymptomatic postmenopausal women will yield about 40 ovarian or adnexal enlargements and fewer than 1 ovarian cancer per 1000 women.[76]

van Nagell and coworkers initiated the use of transvaginal sonography (TVS) at the University of Kentucky 1986 for screening for ovarian cancer.[72,77] They observed that in menstruating women ovarian volume varied markedly throughout the cycle and two-thirds of ovarian enlargements later disappeared. Therefore, they advised that TVS screening be restricted to postmenopausal women who do not have cyclic variation in ovarian volume and who have a higher prevalence of ovarian cancer. They screened 1300 asymptomatic postmenopausal women. Ovarian volume more than 8 cm$^3$ was considered abnormal (width $\times$ height $\times$ thickness $\times$ 0.523) (some use a persistent ovarian tumor volume of 10 cm$^3$ or larger in postmenopausal women as an indication for surgery). This was 2 standard deviations more than the normal postmenopausal ovary. If there was an abnormal volume report, the test was repeated in 4 weeks, and if the ovary was still enlarged, exploratory laparotomy was advised. Ovarian enlargement was found in 33 cases, or 2.5%, although only one-third of these were palpable on physical examina-

tion. Of the 27 patients who had surgery, 14 had ovarian serous cystadenomas; 3 had ovarian carcinomas, of which 1 had a metastatic ovarian carcinoma from an asymptomatic colon carcinoma and 2 had primary ovarian cancers. The latter two had stage Ia disease, negative physical examination, and normal serum Ca 125 tests. Thus, about 63% of those who had a laparotomy had either an ovarian serous cystadenoma or ovarian carcinoma; however, about 37% had unnecessary surgery. Thus TVS had a sensitivity of 1000, a specificity of 0.981, and a positive predictive value of 0.111. These authors' analysis of various studies suggested that TVS is the most reliable technique for screening for ovarian cancer and especially for the discovery of small tumors. Unfortunately, like abdominal ultrasound, TVS has only moderate specificity and positive predictive value. Therefore, it should be combined with other sonography techniques such as morphology index and Doppler flow, and, ideally, with analysis of serum markers.[72]

van Nagell and coworkers observe that in reported 8000 asymptomatic women screened with abdominal or vaginal sonography in their literature review, 10 primary ovarian cancers were discovered, all with stage I disease, and all were cured.[72,77]

Ultrasound screening for familial ovarian cancer was reported by Bourne and the London group.[54] They used transabdominal and transvaginal ultrasound to screen 776 self-referred, asymptomatic women with at least one first-degree (87%) or second-degree (13%) relative with ovarian cancer. The mean age was 51, and most were between 40 and 59. Those with abnormal scans were rescanned from 3 to 8 weeks later to detect size reduction. Both transabdominal and transvaginal scans detected all abnormalities. Positive screening was found in 5.5% (43) of women, who were than referred for surgery. Of 39 women who had a laparotomy, 37 had abnormal ovaries. There was a 48% incidence of bilateral ovarian masses, and 15% of abnormal ovaries had more than one type of pathologic lesion. There were 23 ovarian neoplasms and 32 "tumorlike" conditions, the latter mainly in the premenopausal group. There were 3 well-differentiated primary ovarian cancers, all stage Ia.

Two of the women in the London study were premenopausal—a 38-year-old with a serous cystadenocarcinoma and a 54-year-old with a borderline cystadenoma. One was postmenopausal (63) with a previous hysterectomy and had an endometrioid ovarian carcinoma. The first had a family history of site-specific ovarian cancer. The second had a second-degree relative with ovarian cancer. The third had a first-degree relative with ovarian cancer, but the pedigree suggested a sporadic pattern.

Thus, the ultrasound screening in the London study

had an apparent detection rate (or sensitivity) of 100%. The false-positive rate was 5.2% (40/773), but this was divided into 4% for pre- and postmenopausal women and 10.6% after hysterectomy. The specificity was 94.8%, and the positive predictive value was 7.7%. The prevalence of cancer was 3/776, or 3.9/1000.

The chance of a positive screen's showing any ovarian mass was 19 to 1 (19 masses per 20 laparotomies), the chance of showing any ovarian neoplasm was 1 to 1 (1 neoplasm per 2 laparotomies), and the chance of showing primary ovarian cancer was 1 cancer per 13 laparotomies. The latter is also 12 to 1 odds against finding cancer.

Separate from the three cases discovered by screening scanning was a 55-year-old postmenopausal woman who 8 months after a normal scan had symptoms of disseminated peritoneal adenocarcinoma with apparently normal ovaries. Thus, some cases of stage III disease may be cancer developing at several peritoneal areas simultaneously.

Compared to their corresponding study of asymptomatic, self-referred women from the general population,[73,74] those with familial ovarian cancer had an increased amount of benign and malignant ovarian disease, "and the data are consistent with the hypothesis that some benign tumors may become malignant."[54] The general population group had 11% bilateral masses, while the familial cancer group had 48%. The former had 3% abnormal ovaries with more than one type of pathologic lesion compared with 15% in the latter. The former had a 0.7% incidence of benign epithelial tumor, while the latter had 2.6%. The former had a prevalence of ovarian cancer of 0.4/1000 while the latter had 3.9/1000, or a 10-fold risk increase.

The authors suggest that some benign tumors may become malignant. This is a nontraditional concept. It may affect clinical practice and should encourage research on benign tumors. It is also possible that the malignant ovarian tumors might represent a general tendency toward tumor formation both benign and malignant.

An astonishing incidence of 14.8% small, simple ovarian cysts was reported in 22 of 149 asymptomatic postmenopausal women![78] This unexpected finding was probably due to the combined use of both transabdominal (transpelvic) and transvaginal ultrasound scanning, prospectively done, with a lengthy 30 minutes per examination. All but 2 cysts of the 22 were smaller than 3 cm. Most were identified in only 1 scan view, and only in 6 were both views positive. There was no association with hormone replacement therapy or length of menopause. "The postmenopausal ovary is far more active than has been previously supposed."[78] The cause of cyst formation is unknown.

The first report of a multimodal prospective screening of 1010 apparently healthy postmenopausal women was reported in 1988 from the London Hospital.[79] The reason for the study was that all single techniques of screening lack acceptable specificity. The initial screening was by vaginal examination and measurement of levels of serum Ca 125; abdominal ultrasonography was done as a secondary procedure in selected cases. One cancer was discovered, which was 10 cm and was stage Ia. Thus, in this small series, there was 100% specificity when the three tests were combined. The specificity of serum Ca 125 levels alone was 97.0%, and that of vaginal examinations alone was 97.3%. There were 10 other women who had surgery for nonmalignant conditions. Six had "benign ovarian cysts" at laparotomy. These were not further identified by ultrasound or by pathologic examination as benign neoplasms or simple cysts. The authors wrote, "In the absence of convincing evidence that benign ovarian cysts have pre-malignant potential, vaginal examination and ultrasound scanning either alone or in combination are not acceptable as screening tests for ovarian cancer."[79] Vaginal examination lacks sensitivity. These authors reported a false-positive scan due to adhesions of fluid-filled loops of bowel and a fimbrial cyst. The best choice of an upper limit of Ca 125 screening was between 23 and 30 U/ml. Above this, there is only a little increase in specificity, and below this there is a loss of sensitivity. This limit would result in between 3 to 10% of women being recalled for a second test. Although the results of this study were disappointing, "The combination of serum Ca 125 measurement with ultrasound examination offers the most hope of a specific and sensitive method for the early detection of ovarian cancer."[79]

## ULTRASOUND TO DIFFERENTIATE BENIGN FROM MALIGNANT NEOPLASMS

Ultrasound imaging of ovarian tumor morphology has been used to estimate the probability of malignancy in an already-discovered tumor and is based generally on the amount of echogenic structure in a tumor, except for the characteristic benign dermoid, which usually has solid portions. "However, it has not been possible to find any 100% specific ultrasound criteria for a malignant ovarian tumor except that it is usually complex in its ultrasound appearance."[80]

Timor-Tritsch and colleagues at Columbia University in New York City devised a morphologic scoring system for the differentiation of benign versus malignant ovarian and pelvic lesions using high-frequency real-time transvaginal ultrasonography (see Table 1-1).[81]

**Table 1-1** Transvaginal ultrasound morphology of a new scoring system to predict ovarian malignancy used at Columbia University College of Physicians and Surgeons

| Score Value | Inner Wall Structure | Wall Thickness (mm) | Septa (mm) | Echogenicity |
|---|---|---|---|---|
| 1 | Smooth | Thin (≤3 mm) | No septa | Sonolucent |
| 2 | Irregularities ≤3 mm | Thick (>3 mm) | Thin (≤3 mm) | Low |
| 3 | Papillarities >3 mm | Not applicable, mostly solid | Thick (>3 mm) | Low with echogenic core |
| 4 | Not applicable, mostly solid | | | Mixed |
| 5 | | | | High |
| Maximum | 4 | 3 | 3 | 5 |

SOURCE: Sassone et al.[81]

The system was based on inner wall structure (smooth, irregularities under 3 mm, papillarities over 3 mm, mostly solid), wall thickness (thin under 3 mm, mostly solid), septa (none, thin under 3 mm, thick more than 3 mm), and echogenicity (sonolucent, low echogenicity with echogenic core, mixed echogenicity, high echogenicity). An arbitrary score was assigned for each characteristic, with 1 being the most benign (smooth, thin, no septa, and sonolucent) and 3 to 5 the most malignant. A cutoff score of 9 was found to be the best to distinguish between benign and malignant ovarian neoplasms. In 143 patients with a palpable mass or pain, among whom 20 ovarian malignancies were found, the system had a specificity of 83%, sensitivity of 100%, positive predictive value of 37%, and negative predictive value of 100%. None of the 29 simple cysts were malignant. The threshold may be changed, so that using 10 would make it less sensitive but more specific. Although others consider tumor size to be a risk factor, these authors did not find that size improved sensitivity. In fact, because there were many large benign tumors, inclusion of size further decreased specificity. The main reason for false-positive results was the benign teratoma (dermoid cyst); fortunately, however, simple visualization of the scan made the diagnosis in 23 of 24 cases.[81] "This scoring system seems so far to be the most promising."[80]

Granberg and associates of Göteborg, Sweden, devised an ultrasound morphologic macroscopic classification of ovarian tumors as follows:[80,82]

1. Unilocular: no septation, papillary formation or echogenic contents
2. Unilocular—solid: papillary formation, solid parts or echogenic contents
3. Multilocular: one or more septations without solid areas of papillations
4. Multilocular—solid: one or more septations with solid parts, papillary formation or echogenic contents
5. Solid: more than 80% solid-echogenic

The tumor is measured in two perpendicular planes. If the ovarian cyst is larger than 8 cm, endovaginal (transvaginal) ultrasound cannot be relied upon to determine whether the cyst is unilocular or multilocular. Transabdominal ultrasound is needed to view the upper part of the cyst for septations and echogenic areas when the unilocular cyst is 2 to 3 cm larger than the focal range of the endovaginal transducer. Granberg and colleagues found that 96% of their ultrasound images agreed with the macroscopic characterization of the pathologist. There was one malignancy in a unilocular 5-cm ovarian cyst. In retrospect, "it contained some macroscopically visible papillary formations and should thus probably have been classified as unilocular-solid by endovaginal ultrasound."[80] Although increasing size is associated with increasing chance of malignancy in other enlargements, this is not true for the unilocular cyst. The chance of malignancy increases with complexity, size, and age. There is about an 18% chance of malignancy in complex cysts.

The percentage chance of malignancy in unilocular cysts was 0.3%, in unilocular solid tumors it was 2%, in multilocular solid tumors it was 36%, and in solid tumors it was 39%. The most frequent structure in malignant tumors was papillary vegetation on the cyst wall.[80,82]

In a series of 100 women undergoing laparotomy for ovarian masses, the sonographic diagnosis was correct in 68%. Of 30 cancers, 24 were identified, giving a sensitivity of 80%.

The positive predictive value for malignancy was 73%, and the negative predictive value for excluding a malignancy was 91%.[83]

The University of Kentucky group devised a transvaginal ultrasound morphology index based on volume, cyst wall structure, and septa structure (see Table 1-2).[84] Ovarian tumors less than 15 cm in diameter were evaluated in 64 premenopausal and 57 postmenopausal women. There were 12 malignant and 109 benign tumors. In the premenopausal group, the mean morphology score of benign tumors was 4.12 ± 0.34, while the

**Table 1-2** Transvaginal ultrasound morphology index of ovarian tumors used at University of Kentucky

|   | Volume (cm³) | Cyst Wall Structure | Septa |
|---|---|---|---|
| 0 | <10 | Smooth <3 mm thickness | None |
| 1 | 10–50 | Smooth >3 mm thickness | Thin (<3 mm) |
| 2 | >50–200 | Papillary projection <3 mm | Thick 3 mm–1 cm |
| 3 | >200–500 | Papillary projection ≥3 mm | Solid area ≥1 cm |
| 4 | >500 | Predominantly solid | Predominantly solid |

SOURCE: DePriest et al.[84]

malignant tumors were 8.0 ± 0.45. In the postmenopausal group, the benign tumor score was 2.94 ± 0.28 while the malignant score was 8.22 ± 0.42. Overall there were no malignancies with a morphology index less than 5. This may increase the specificity of transvaginal ultrasound.[84]

A normal-sized ovary carcinoma syndrome that may have normal diagnostic imaging has been described.[85] Such cases might be primary serous cystadenocarcinoma of the peritoneum.

It is generally recognized that the postmenopausal ovary is smaller than that of the menstruating woman. Until recently it was assumed that the postmenopausal ovary is dormant. Indeed, palpation of a normal-size premenstrual ovary in a postmenopausal woman is a cause for concern, and a cystic enlargement has been an appropriate indication for surgery. Subsequently, it was found that most small postmenopausal ovarian cysts are not malignant, and therefore there has been a high incidence of "false-positive" ultrasound scans.

Levine and associates reported combined transabdominal and transvaginal ultrasound examinations in 184 asymptomatic postmenopausal volunteers.[86] They found an astonishing 17% with simple adnexal cysts at the initial examination! There were 37 cysts in 32 women. The ultrasound examinations were repeated every 3 months for 1 year and then every 6 months during the second year. It was found that these simple cysts (completely anechoic, unilocular, nonseptated cysts) were amazingly dynamic. Forty-six new cysts appeared in 31 women, 11 of whom previously had cysts. Of 49 women with 72 cysts with subsequent scanning, 38 (or 50%) of the 72 cysts disappeared completely, 20 (or 28%) remained constant in size, 8 (or 11%) enlarged, 2 (or 3%) decreased in size, and 4 (or 6%) both increased and decreased in size.

Thus, the previous concept of a high "false-positive" rate has to be redefined in that the simple cyst is usually found to be benign.[86] The high incidence in this study was due to the combined used of both the transabdominal and transvaginal route, since small cysts are easily missed by only one route. Most cysts were 1 cm. Only 7 cysts were 3 cm or larger. The largest was 4.7 cm and subsequently disappeared. Six women had surgery. One had a 4-cm ultrasonically simple cyst that was operated upon because of the "unusually large" size and was found to be a papillary serous cystadenoma. Two patients had complex masses; one mass was a dermoid cyst (2.2 cm) and one was a stage Ic ovarian carcinoma (4 cm with an abnormal resistive index). Three with septated cysts had two hydrosalpinges and one distal tubal cyst. The cancer patient had had a normal sonography 15 months previously (and had a normal pelvic examination and Ca 125 test). The authors comment, "It remains uncertain whether the presence of ovarian cysts in menopausal women is a risk factor for ovarian carcinoma."[86] Ovarian cysts were investigated by morphology (simple cyst; septated cyst; complex cyst with more than two septations or solid elements; and solid lesions), and by color Doppler resistive index (RI). The cysts normal value was over 0.7, indicating a high distal resistance. The authors advised that in postmenopausal women, simple adnexal cysts less than 3 cm in greatest diameter with a normal RI and a normal Ca 125 test are most likely benign and may be observed safely with ultrasound. They advised surgical resection for larger cysts, those with unusual nodules or septations, and those with Doppler prominent diastolic flow.[86]

These authors did not find an association of cysts with hormone replacement therapy or duration of menopause.[86]

The above findings raise questions with profound implications. Why does the postmenopausal ovary have a relatively high incidence of dynamic small simple cyst formation? Why has this not been reported by pathologists? Is it a new phenomenon or has it simply been overlooked or not reported? Do these apparently functional dynamic simple cysts have any relation to later formulation of ovarian cancer? If a cyst persists is it a true neoplasm, such as a serous cystadenoma? Do such neoplasms become malignant? Should they be removed even if they do not become malignant?

The clinical significance is that with ultrasound, postmenopausal small unilocular cystic enlargements of the ovary have been discovered to be not rare, and most postmenopausal ovarian cysts are not malignant. Granberg and Wikland found 1 case of malignancy in 140 simple cysts.[80] Their literature review found 11 malignancies (2.9%) associated with 373 benign unilocular cysts by transabdominal ultrasound, and no malignancies in 146 cases of unilocular anechoid cysts discovered by endovaginal ultrasound. They feel that because transabdominal ultrasound is not as reliable as transvaginal ultrasound in detecting cyst echogenic contents, a larger amount of echogenic material would have to be present for positive transabdominal scans. Therefore, positive transabdominal scans would tend to have a higher percentage chance of malignancy than positive transvaginal scans.

Since most small unilocular cysts in postmenopausal women are benign, how should they be managed? Various approaches have been suggested, and there are many differences of opinion.[80]

1. If the cyst is 5 cm or less and asymptomatic, serial ultrasound examinations are done at 1, 3, 6, and 12 months. If the cyst enlarges or becomes echogenic or becomes symptomatic, it is removed.
2. Laparoscopic removal of the cyst is performed.
3. Transvaginal ultrasound–guided needle aspiration of the cyst is done.
4. The cyst is removed after 1 year to avoid potential malignant change.
5. Laparotomy removal of the cyst is performed.

Needle aspiration is very controversial.[87] About 70% are cured with just one puncture. Cytologic examination of aspirated fluid is not reliable. If the cyst recurs, there is a 60% chance that surgery will be required eventually. Neoplastic cysts will recur. This implies that most unilocular cysts are not neoplastic. Experimentally, some clinicians have aspirated cysts and replaced the contents with 95% alcohol for 5 minutes to reduce the recurrence rate to 7%.

Separate from the issue of screening for ovarian cancer is the question of how to manage the discovered small unilocular cystic ovarian mass, since most will not be malignant. Prior to the use of ultrasound, the traditional chance that surgery for an ovarian tumor in a postmenopausal woman would yield a malignant result was close to 50%. Sonograms have a high incidence of false-positives. "The emergence of pelvic ultrasound has increased the rate of intervention for ovarian neoplasms, resulting in rates of only one malignancy per 33 operations."[88] This tends to reduce enthusiasm for laparotomy removal of the apparently benign small cystic ovary.

The role of laparoscopy in management of ovarian cysts and tumors is controversial.

If the enlarged ovary appears benign by

1. Physical examination (cystic, no solid parts)
2. TVS (unilateral; cystic; unilocular or thin septa; no internal papillations or excrescences; no solid areas; no ascites; no matted bowel)
3. Serum Ca 125 testing

and if the patient gives informed consent, then laparoscopic surgery may be considered because of a low risk of ovarian malignancy. Aside from the small unilocular cystic ovary, on an experimental basis, some remove presumably benign ovarian neoplasms.

At laparoscopy the abdomen is inspected for ascites and excrescences of the surface of the ovary. Washing and aspiration is done with normal saline including under the diaphragm. Large cysts are aspirated by needle and then with a wider suction tube. The entire ovarian cyst is removed for frozen section. Any spill is treated by irrigation with distilled water to lyse any cancer cells. The opposite ovary is removed in postmenopausal women. Frozen section is done on the cyst wall. Cyst fluid cytologic examination is not reliable. If malignancy is discovered, then an immediate staging laparotomy is done.

The advantage is the removal of benign ovarian cysts and cystic neoplasms with a minimum of surgery, especially in elderly postmenopausal women.

The disadvantage is that no large series has been studied for long-term follow-up and to know whether spillage of an early ovarian cancer will worsen the prognosis. Seeding of the abdominal laparoscopy tract by cancer has occurred. Finally, even with standard TVS that shows a benign cyst, unexpectedly a malignancy may be discovered.

In a group of 1011 premenopausal woman who had a laparoscopy for an adnexal mass, unexpectedly, four were found to have ovarian cancer.[89] Three had been treated for endometriosis. Vaginal ultrasonography was not reliable because complex masses can be produced by endometriomas, benign cystic teratomas, and intraligamentous myomas. Neither serum Ca 125 levels, age, cyst size, nor peritoneal cytology was reliable. Simple aspiration of an ovarian cyst was considered inadequate. Adequate biopsies and cyst wall pathologic examination were necessary. A laparoscopy bag, copious irrigation, and removal of tissue, sometimes by colpotomy, were used. Despite spillage and despite the delay in oncology laparotomy, the authors thought that no harm was done (although follow-up was inadequate). It is interesting that the ages of the patients varied from 33 to 45 and that they had fertility problems and endometriosis. Family history was not given, and these cases may have been early-onset familial ovarian cancer associated with infertility.

Radiologists feel that single unilocular simple ovarian cysts up to 5 cm in postmenopausal women are almost always benign.[90] Even up to 10 cm, simple cysts are usually benign.

Serous cystadenomas tend to be cystic and thin-walled, with thin septa and no or few internal echoes. Serous cystic cystadenocarcinomas tend to have more internal architecture; multiple septa; increased echogenicity; papillary projections and vegetation; focal areas of irregular mural thickening; loss of wall definition; fixation to surrounding structures; ascites; and omental caking.

Mucinous cystadenocarcinomas tend to have even more solid elements.

Solid ovarian neoplasms may be germ cell tumors, Brenner tumors, or thecomas.

Metastases to the ovary may have a complex cystic mass with solid components and may have come from the breast or gastrointestinal tract. Solid areas may result from lymphoma and leukemia.

Dermoid cysts (benign mature cystic teratomas) have a characteristic appearance with echogenic solid areas.

Multilocular cysts have about an 8% chance of being malignant, multilocular-solid tumors have about a 70% chance of malignancy, and solid tumors have about a 40% chance of malignancy.[90] With ovarian cancer only about 70% of morphologic ultrasonography may indicate malignancy. The sensitivity is about 70 to 80%, and the specificity about 90%. In about 10 to 15%, morphology alone cannot distinguish benign from malignant tumors.

## TRANSVAGINAL ULTRASOUND COLOR FLOW AND DOPPLER WAVE ANALYSIS

Aside from determining transvaginal ultrasound ovarian tumor morphology, color Doppler flow analysis was developed to help differentiate benign ovarian neoplasms and masses from malignant ovarian neoplasms. The purpose was to reduce false-positive reports and increase diagnostic accuracy.

Contrary to conventional thought, color Doppler flow is not usually used for screening. Screening is done by transabdominal and transvaginal ultrasonography. Screening of the general population is not standard practice. Color Doppler flow has been used only if an abnormality is discovered. Without fanfare and almost without realization, in communities where it is available, color Doppler flow examination has become standard practice to study already-discovered ovarian tumors. This concept is not generally appreciated.

I have discovered an interesting controversy about who first used transvaginal color flow imaging to differentiate benign versus malignant ovarian neoplasms.

In 1992, Professor Asim Kurjak of the University of Zagreb, Yugoslavia, cited his earliest reference, Transvaginal color Doppler for the assessment of pelvic circulation, published in 1989:[92] "Kurjak et al. were the first to report that transvaginal color flow imaging can be

used in the assessment of pelvic circulation and to differentiate between benign and malignant pelvic tumors."[91] He also said in 1992, "Diagnosis of ovarian carcinoma at an early stage was very unusual before color Doppler ultrasound was introduced by us in 1987 for examination of the pelvic organs."[91]

Bourne, Campbell, Steer, et al. of King's College School of Medicine, London, in their 1989 publication *Transvaginal colour flow imaging: A possible new screening technique for ovarian cancer,* wrote, "To the best of our knowledge, this is the first report that transvaginal color flow imaging can be used to differentiate between primary ovarian cancer and many forms of benign pelvic masses."[93]

Although reports from both groups were published in the same year, since Professor Kurjak had studied ultrasonography with Professor Stuart Campbell in London, since the London group had already done original work in transabdominal screening for ovarian cancer as well as Doppler flow in pregnancy, since the London paper dealt specifically with ovarian tumors, and since the London paper had the greater impact, it is assumed by most that Bourne and Campbell were the first to do the work.

Nevertheless, both groups are world leaders in this field, with great experience and expertise. Furthermore, good ideas spontaneously develop in different places simultaneously, especially with the fertilizing medical tradition of sharing new concepts. The bottom line is that we all benefit by their pioneer work.

Color Doppler flow analysis is based on the neovascularity of malignant tumors.[95] The pioneer in this field is Folkman, who found in cancers an angiogenesis factor that induces proliferation of endothelial cells.[94] Cancers cannot enlarge more than 2 to 3 mm without neovascularity.[95] New cancer tumor vessels develop from older preexisting normal vessels that have the usual uniform distribution and structure of arterioles with endothelium, with smooth muscle wall media, and with an external adventia. The new cancer tumor vessels have no or very little smooth muscle wall media and are bizarre endothelial-linked spaces with adventitia. They are irregular in distribution, tortuous, dilated, and amorphous and have sinusoidal blood lakes and arteriovenous shunts. Thus, the cancer vessels have a reduced resistance to blood flow, have an increased blood flow and blood volume, and have turbulent flow.[95] Ultrasound color flow can detect abnormal blood vessels as small as 1 mm in diameter if the velocity is greater than 1 cm/s.[96] "Most normal cells do not secrete angiogenetic substances except during embryogenesis, growth, wound repair, or formation of corpus luteum."[93]

Doppler flow measurements may be misleading in premenopausal women with newly growing blood vessels without muscular walls such as in the corpus luteum, or with pelvic inflammatory disease. Therefore, scanning should be done in the proliferative phase.

In general, with transvaginal ultrasonography the ovarian tumor is first imaged to determine its size and internal macroscopic anatomy. Suspicious ovarian signs include papillations, septa, solid areas, and capsule thickening. Suspicious signs outside of the ovary include ascites and metastases to the omentum and liver. Following this, color flow imaging is done.

Color imaging uses two-dimensional, real-time display of blood flow information.[97] The presence of color with its hues, saturations, and brightness is superimposed on the two-dimensional gray-scale ultrasound image. Such color shows the presence of blood flow, direction toward the transducer (red) or away from the transducer (blue), speed, and type of flow (laminar, disturbed, turbulent). *Hue* refers to the color. *Saturation* refers to the concentration of the color. *Brightness* refers to the amount of light in the color.

Color flow shows more readily with large volume and rapid rate of flow, which tends to occur in malignant neoplasms as does turbulent and irregular flow. Without color flow, it would be difficult to identify small vessels for pulsed Doppler velocity waveform study. The vessels may be in the surface periphery or in the central area.

After color signals are located over blood vessels, the sample volume range gate is used to activate the pulsed Doppler and record blood flow velocity waveforms over the colored vessels from the wall, septum, and solid areas or echogenic core. Several measurements are made of each area, and the lowest values are used.

The Doppler shift signal is a waveform created by circulating red blood cells during one cadiac cycle. Cells going toward the transducer cause upward displacement of the baseline, while those cells going away cause a downward shift of the baseline. Although velocity and volume of flow cannot be measured precisely, resistance to flow can be studied.

The amplitude of the Doppler shift measures the ratio of the systolic to diastolic blood flow. The shape of the curve depends on the incident angle of the ultrasound beam. At small angles, the waveforms are peaked. As the angle increases, the waveform becomes rounded, and finally at 90 degrees (perpendicular to the vessel) there is no Doppler shift and no waveform is produced.

The simplest method of calculating resistance is the S/D ratio (developed in 1980),[98] or the ratio of the peak systolic to the end diastolic shifts. A decreasing ratio indicates decreasing downstream resistance and increased diastolic flow.

The pulsatility index (PI) was developed in 1975.[98] It is the peak systolic flow minus the end diastolic flow divided by the mean, or $(S - D)/\text{mean}$.

The resistance index (RI) was devised in 1974.[98] It is the peak systolic flow minus the end diastolic flow divided by the peak systolic flow, or $(S - D)/S$ (see Fig. 1-1).

All the above Doppler indices decrease with increased diastolic blood flow.

Different authors use different indices.[98] The London group (Stuart Campbell) uses the PI, with which benign tumors generally have a value over 1 with a range of 3.2 to 7.0, while malignant tumors usually have a value less than 1 with a range of 0.3 to 1.0.[93]

The Zagreb, Yugoslavia, group (Kurjak) uses an RI, with which benign tumors tend to have a value greater than 0.40, while malignant ones have a lower value (0.25 to 0.40).[88]

The group at Nagoya University, Japan (Kawai), uses the reciprocal of the PI (1/PI), with which benign disease has a value less than 0.8 (mean $0.69 \pm 0.05$) while malignant disease has a value greater than 0.8 ($1.87 \pm 0.65$).[99]

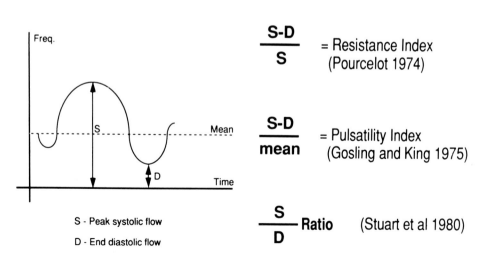

$$\frac{S-D}{S} = \text{Resistance Index (Pourcelot 1974)}$$

$$\frac{S-D}{\text{mean}} = \text{Pulsatility Index (Gosling and King 1975)}$$

$$\frac{S}{D}\ \text{Ratio} \quad (\text{Stuart et al 1980})$$

S - Peak systolic flow

D - End diastolic flow

**Fig. 1-1** Qualitative methods for waveform analysis. From Meyer WJ, Jaffe R, Basic principles of Doppler ultrasonography, in *Color Doppler Imaging in Obstetrics and Gynecology*, Jaffe R, Warsof SL, eds, New York, McGraw-Hill, 1992, p 13.

Transabdominal pulsed Doppler imaging can show blood flow in major vessels. Color Doppler TVS can show small vessel circulation or capillary "blush."

Doppler waveform study of tumors shows an increase in signal amplitude due to more moving red blood cells, an increase in peak systole flow, and high diastolic shift reduces the systolic-diastolic Doppler waveform variation.

The first report of transvaginal color flow imaging, *Transvaginal colour flow imaging: A possible new screening technique for ovarian cancer,*[93] had an error in the title. It was not for screening purposes; rather it was to differentiate benign from malignant ovarian neoplasms. This confusion of purpose has been perpetuated in the literature.

In this first study, 20 women were selected because of previous transvaginal ultrasound scanning that showed abnormal morphology and/or volume, and there were 30 controls.[93] Premenopausal women were scanned during cycle days 1 to 8 to avoid corpus luteum neovascularization. Neovascularization was recognized by prominent color with "continuously fluctuating colour rather than the pulsatile colour seen with normal arteries."[93] This would indicate large flow volumes through many small and/or passively dilated vessels. Another feature was used: Doppler flow velocity waveforms. The transducer angle was adjusted to obtain the maximum waveforms amplitude. The authors decided to use a PI to quantitate results. PI calculated electronically averaging three cardiac cycles was peak systolic Doppler shift frequency (A) minus maximum end diastolic Doppler shift frequency (B) divided by the mean maximum Doppler shift frequency over the cardiac cycle (mean). In normal ovaries, the PI increases with distal vascular bed constriction. With cancer, there should be a low PI due to decreased impedance to flow in the distal vessels. The lowest PI values were from ovaries in which a specific blood vessel could not be identified. Aside from color flow and measurement of PI, ovarian size and morphology were rechecked. In the 30 normal controls and 2 patients with hydrosalpinges (presumably old), there was no neovascularization and the PI ranged from 3.1 to 9.4. Benign tumors (9 patients) also did not show neovascularization and had a PI of 3.2 to 7.0, which values were slightly lower than those of the normal controls. One patient with bilateral dermoid cysts with thyroid cells had neovascularization and PIs of 0.4 and 0.8. Of the 20 patients with masses, 7 had primary ovarian cancer that showed "clear evidence of neovascularization," with PIs from 0.3 to 1.0. Two were stage Ia, four were stage III, and one was stage IV. One patient with an intraepithelial serous cystadenocarcinoma in a small ovary had no vascular change and a PI of 5.5.

Kurjak and associates examined 14,317 women (87% premenopausal) with abdominal color-pulsed Doppler scanning.[91] The RI was calculated from five separate cardiac cycles and the mean recorded. In premenopausal women, sonography was done on days 3 to 10 of the menstrual cycle to avoid the corpus luteum increased blood flow. Among 8620 asymptomatic women and 5697 women with a suspected adnexal mass, 624 benign adnexal tumors were diagnosed by laparotomy. In all but one, the RI was greater than 0.40. There were 60 malignant ovarian tumors discovered. Among stage I ovarian cancers discovered, there were 11 primary and 9 secondary tumors, all between 3.5 and 5 cm. Of the primary neoplasms, 5 were in women with a known mass and 6 were in the asymptomatic group. In 9 of the 11 primary cancers, neovascularization was found with an RI of 0.32 to 0.40. In the 9 secondary cancers, the RI range was 0.28 to 0.40 and there was less prominent color. In 5 of these 9 metastatic cancers, there was no abnormality on clinical examination or on transabdominal or simple B-mode transvaginal ultrasound. (If this is confirmed, it means that metastatic ovarian cancer can be identified by color Doppler transvaginal ultrasound before it enlarges the ovary and before it is found on routine transvaginal ultrasound. This is a significant finding and suggests that microscopic malignant neoplasms cause neovascularization.) The other 40 cancers were stage III and IV, with 39 showing characteristic Doppler flow. Three were asymptomatic. The RI sensitivity was 90.8%, specificity 99.4%, positive predictive value 93.6%, negative predictive value 99.1%, and accuracy 98.6%. Kurjak and associates developed a scoring system, the Zagreb ultrasound and Doppler scoring system for adnexal masses, based on morphology, color flow, and RI (see Fig. 1-2). Using their scoring system for 5 cancers found in 1623 women, when an RI cutoff point of only 0.4 was used, there were 2 true-positives, 3 false-negatives, and 3 false-positives. With the whole scoring system cutoff point of 4 or more, there were positive diagnoses in all 5 cancers, false-positives in 4, and no false-negatives. The false-positives were pelvic inflammatory disease or corpus luteum neovascularization.

Timor-Tritsch and associates combined their transvaginal ultrasound morphometric scoring system with color flow to locate blood vessels and then did Doppler blood flow velocity waveform measurements on ovarian tumors to distinguish between previously discovered benign and malignant tumors scheduled for surgery.[100] Of 16 malignant ovarian tumors, all were detected by either high morphometric scoring or low flow resistance, or both, while 78 benign tumors were identified by low morphometric scoring and/or high resistance to flow. All 14 masses with a high total score

**Ovarian tumor ultrasound—Doppler classification**
**(Circle characteristics seen and add for score.)**

Patient name _____   Date _____   Institution _____

| | Fluid | | Internal borders | | Size |
|---|---|---|---|---|---|
| Unilocular | Clear | (0) | Smooth | (0) | |
| | Internal echoes | (1) | Irregular | (2) | |
| Multilocular | Clear | (1) | Smooth | (1) | |
| | Internal echoes | (1) | Irregular | (2) | |
| Cystic-solid | Clear | (1) | Smooth | (1) | |
| | Internal echoes | (2) | Irregular | (2) | |
| Papillary projections | Suspicious | (1) | Definite | (2) | |
| Solid | Homogenous | (1) | Echogenic | (2) | |
| Peritoneal fluid | Absent | (0) | Present | (1) | |

| Color Doppler | | | RI (index) | | Velocity |
|---|---|---|---|---|---|
| No vessels seen | | (0) | (0) | | |
| Regular separate vessels | | (1) | >0.40 | (1) | |
| Randomly dispersed vessels | | (2) | <0.41 | (2) | |

If suspected corpus luteum, repeat in next menstrual cycle in proliferative phase.

| Score | Ultrasound | Color |
|---|---|---|
| < 2 | Benign | Benign |
| 3–4 | Questionable | Questionable |
| > 4 | Suspicious | |

**Fig. 1-2** The Zagreb ultrasound and Doppler scoring system for adnexal masses. From Kurjak A, Zalud I, Ultrasound assessment of adnexal masses, in *Color Doppler Imaging in Obstetrics and Gynecology,* Jaffe R, Warsof SL, eds, New York, McGraw-Hill, 1992, p 280.

and low RI or PI had malignancies. All 67 masses with a low morphology score and a high RI or PI were benign. The score of 8 resulted in 1 malignancy's being overlooked, but it was correctly identified by a low RI (0.44) and low PI (0.6). One malignancy was overlooked by a high RI (0.56) and high PI (0.8) but was identified by a high morphology score of 12.

Inflammatory adnexities and the corpus luteum show angiogenesis or vessel dilatation.

In the study of Timor-Tritsch and colleagues, the mean total score (morphologic and color flow–directed Doppler) for benign masses was 6.7 (range 4 to 12) and for malignant masses was 11.7 (range 8 to 14).[100] The RI was 0.64 (range 0.23 to 0.98) for benign tumors and 0.39 for malignant tumors with a range of 0.2 to 0.53. The mean PI of benign tumors was 1.17 (range 0.27 to 2.6) and of malignancies was 0.52 (range 0.2 to 0.8). There was no cancer if no color flow was obtained. "In general, malignant masses exhibited flow patterns with increased velocity and areas of turbulent flow."[100] The morphologic scoring system alone had a sensitivity of 94%, specificity of 87%, and positive predictive value of 60%. With either RI or PI, the sensitivity was 94%,

specificity 99%, and positive predictive value 94%. Among the 16 malignant tumors were 4 of LMP that tested like malignancy. Five hydrosalpinges and tubo-ovarian complexes correctly tested benign and presumably were old and quiescent. The authors found that the cutoff points resulting in the best differentiation of benign versus malignant in series were RI 0.46 and PI 0.62, with higher values being benign and lower values being malignant.

In another study, preoperative transvaginal color flow imaging was done for 53 persistent ovarian masses, of which 36 were benign and 17 were malignant.[101] It was more reliable than simple ultrasound morphology or serum Ca 125 levels. In 16 of the 17 malignant cases, there were intratumoral blood vessels with low impedence to flow and a PI always below 1. Among 36 benign tumors, 35 had a PI of over 1, although 11 had suspicious sonographic morphology and 14 had elevated serum Ca 125 levels. The sensitivity and specificity of PI in detection of malignancy were 94 and 97%; in detection of suspicious sonographic morphology, 94 and 69%; and in detection of elevated serum Ca 125 levels, 82 and 61%. "More over, because early development of neovascularity may precede tumor growth, screening for ovarian malignancy with transvaginal color flow imaging may detect early ovarian neoplasms before (simple morphology) sonography.''[101]

Although color Doppler ultrasound has not been used for initial screening programs, recent research has suggested that early ovarian malignancy may have abnormal color Doppler findings before morphologic abnormalities are detectable with standard transvaginal ultrasound.[91,101] Therefore, if high-risk cases were to be screened, it would be appropriate to consider color Doppler transvaginal ultrasound.

In a Nagoya University report on a group of 24 women with ovarian masses, 15 of the masses were benign and 9 were malignant.[99] The reciprocal of the PI (1/PI) was $0.69 \pm 0.05$ in benign tumors and $1.87 \pm 0.65$ in malignant tumors. With a cutoff value of 1/PI set at 0.8 (corresponding to a cut off of PI of 1.25), 23 of 24 were identified correctly, giving an accuracy of 95.8%. Among 11 tumors with a low Ca 125 level, all 5 malignant tumors had a high 1/PI (above 0.8) and all benign tumors had a low 1/PI or nondetectable waveforms. There were 10 cases with a benign morphologic appearance, of which 1 in fact was malignant. Of 14 cases with a malignant morphologic appearance, 8 were malignant and 6 were benign. One of the malignant cases was a mucinous cystadenoma of low-grade malignancy. It had a malignant-type Doppler flow study. Thus color flow Doppler analysis was much more reliable than sonographic morphologic analysis or serum Ca 125 tests.

A Vanderbilt University study showed that with Doppler waveform analysis, benign ovarian neoplasms and masses tend to have a lower maximum systolic-velocity flow (about 2 to 37 cm/s), a high-impedance (low-diastolic) flow with a PI over 1.0, a diastolic notch (between systolic and diastolic), and blood flow at the periphery of the ovarian mass.[96] Malignant tumors tend to have higher maximum systolic velocity (about 5 to 60 cm/s), a low-impedance (high-diastolic) PI less than 1.0, no diastolic notch, and abnormal increased blood flow at the center of the mass.

Low-impedance flow (PI less than 1.0) tends to occur with ovarian cancer but also with benign conditions with neovascularity such as inflammatory masses, metabolically active masses, and corpus luteum cysts.[96]

Intermediate-impedance flow (PI 1.0 to 1.5) tends to occur with dermoid cysts and endometriomas.[96]

High-impedance flow (PI over 1.5) tends to occur with ovarian benign cystadenoma and hemorrhagic cysts.[96]

In a series of 62 cases of surgically removed ovarian masses, there were 25 malignant neoplasms, among which 20 had low-impedance flow (PI less than 1.0) and none had a diastolic notch.[96] Two benign dermoid cysts

and one tubo-ovarian abscess also had a low-impedance blood flow (false-positive malignant). One malignant tumor was incorrectly thought to be benign. The negative predictive value was 98%, while the positive predictive value was only 83%. This means that for every 4 cases with a malignant report, only 3 would be malignant. The sensitivity and specificity in detecting ovarian cancer were 85 and 93%.

Emphasizing studying central rather than peripheral tumor blood vessels, with sonographic morphology combined with color Doppler flow, some have reported a sensitivity of 100%, a specificity of 99.8%, a positive predictive value of 83.5%, and a negative predictive value of 100%.[102]

Kurjak and Predanić devised a new scoring system for prediction of ovarian malignancy using transvaginal morphologic and color Doppler sonography.[103] Transvaginal B mode was used for morphologic analysis based on internal borders, quality of cyst, septations, papillary projections, and ovarian echogenicity. The classification of abnormal ovaries included unilocular and multilocular cystic, cystic-solid, or solid. The dividing line of ovarian enlargement was 9 cm$^3$. Color Doppler flow was used to assess vascular location (pericystic, peripheral, central, septal, papillary projection) and type of neovascularization (no vessel seen, regularly separated vessels, randomly dispersed vessels). Pulsed Doppler waveform analysis of visualized vessels (vascular quality) was used for the RI. RI above 0.4 was considered a benign flow pattern; less than 0.4 was considered malignant. The corpus luteum was avoided in premenopausal patients because of its increased blood flow (see Fig. 1-2).

Using morphologic criteria, of 38 malignant tumors, 3 were erroneously considered benign because there was no septation, papillae, or solid areas.[103] Thus morphologic analysis alone is not reliable.

Even with a cutoff point of 0.40 RI, there was overlap between benign and malignant lesions.[103]

Kurjak and Predanić added and emphasized two new criteria—not found in other scoring systems—vascular location and type of vascularity.[103] Blood flow in septa, papillae, and solid, inhomogeneous areas was considered suspicious. Randomly dispersed vessels seen in a small cross-sectional area of the ovary is also associated with malignancy. (Borderline tumors may not have neovascularization and may not be able to be detected on color flow.) "These should be considered new criteria for screening for ovarian malignancy by transvaginal color Doppler sonography."[103]

These authors reported a sensitivity of 97.3%, a specificity of 100%, a positive predictive value of 100%, a negative predictive value of 99.2%, and accuracy of 97.3%.[103] When only morphologic criteria were used, the sensitivity was 92.1%, the specificity 94.8%, the positive predictive value 79.5%, and the negative predictive value 97.7%.

The authors recommended that "suspicious" (normal morphologic appearance, but with areas of neovascularization) and "malignant"-appearing lesions be operated upon.[103] "Questionable" (suspicious morphologic appearance but no neovascularization) lesions are followed by color Doppler TVS.

Kurjak, Schulman (New York), and associates combined transvaginal B-mode real-time imaging ultrasound, color flow, and Doppler waveform analysis to study adnexal masses in 1000 postmenopausal women.[88] There were 29 malignant neoplasms (35%) in 83 women who had surgery. Morphology alone had poor sensitivity. Color flow was identified in 27 malignancies and in 35% of benign masses. A Doppler resistance index of feeder vessels with a cutoff value of 0.4 gave a sensitivity of 96%, a specificity of 95%, a positive predictive value of 96%, and a negative predictive value of 95%. Color flow was imposed on the tumor to identify feeder vessels. The Doppler cursor was placed on the flashing of each vessel and a flow velocity waveform recorded. The RI was calculated as the systolic peak minus the diastolic trough divided by the systolic peak. Normal pelvic vessels have an RI of 0.8 to 0.5, while abnormal or larger diastolic low-pressure flows have an RI below 0.41. The artery with the lowest RI was used. Although color flow is usually observed in malignant tumors (sensitivity 93%), the specificity was only 65%. Thus Doppler measurements are important.

The 29 malignant ovarian tumors came from a group of 83 patients who had surgery and therefore was compatible with the chance of finding a malignancy in postmenopausal women by clinical evaluation alone prior to the use of ultrasound.[88]

The authors indicate that since the use of ultrasound, others have reported only 1 malignancy per 33 operations, in part because of benign neoplasms.[88]

The authors found a "sharper separation" of Doppler indices than other investigators, which they attributed to "differences in instrument design and settings."[88] They felt that blood flow may vary with "metastatic potential" or stage. It should be noted that in their series of 29 malignant tumors, only 7 were in stage I, and only 4 were asymptomatic. Returning to the question of scanning, they wrote "An important unanswered question is the reliability of transvaginal ultrasound in visualizing the ovary and detecting disease."[104] They suggested that adding simple color flow to scanning transvaginal ultrasound might permit detection of tumors less than 1 cm that would otherwise be missed.[88]

Hata et al. of Shimane University in Japan reported three cases of LMP mucinous ovarian cystadenoma tumors.[104] All had a benign appearance by conventional B-mode sonography, computed tomography, and magnetic reasonance imaging. All had normal serum levels of Ca 125, tissue polypeptide antigen, and carcinoembryonic agent. They were multilocular cystic tumors with thin regular septa and walls without intracystic vegetations. Blood flow velocity waveforms could be detected in the three cases. In 26 benign ovarian tumors, the RI was $0.818 \pm 0.223$ while the 3 cases of LMP had an RI of $0.418 \pm 0.072$. The latter therefore had waveforms of relatively high diastolic flow and low pulsatility, which are usually present in malignant ovarian tumors. Two standard deviations from the LMP tumor RI value of 0.418 is 0.56. Using the latter as a cutoff, all of the 3 LMP tumors and 3 of 26 benign tumors had lower values suggesting malignancy. Thus with the dividing RI line at 0.56, the sensitivity or detection rate for LMP tumors was 100% while the false-positive rate was 11.5%, which occurred in serous cystadenoma, fibroma, and hemorrhagic corpus luteum cyst. The specificity was 88.5%, the predictive value of a positive result was 50.0%, the predictive value of a negative result was 100.0%, and the accuracy was 89.7%. The authors realized that ovulation and corpus luteum activity can affect ovarian arterial compliance and therefore in premenopausal women did the Doppler blood flow velocity waveforms on days 5 to 7 of the menstrual cycle. Thus transvaginal Doppler blood velocity waveform testing is useful in differentiating benign versus LMP ovarian tumors that otherwise have a benign appearance on standard pelvic and transvaginal ultrasound. These authors use a single transvaginal transducer probe that gave a combined B-mode imaging, color, and pulsed Doppler to simultaneously visualize structure and blood flow. The color flow made it easier and faster to locate vessels to sample. The authors reported a surprising finding. In histologic sections of all the 26 benign and 3 LMP tumors, there were endothelial-lined sinusoidal spaces without muscular elements! There were no histologic photographs. "Since the vessels are collapsed in a histologic section, it is difficult to know how large these spaces are in vivo and to detect the significant differences in space size between benign and malignant tumors."[104]

Color Doppler flow suggests that the malignant tumor has larger sinusoids. This is compatible with the tendency of malignant tumors to be friable and hemorrhagic. Perhaps the malignant tumor secretes a more potent or larger amount of tumor angiogenesis factor for a faster growth and/or larger sinusoids. It is interesting that Timor-Tritsch and colleagues had four cases of LMP tumors[100] and Kawai and colleagues[99] had one case, which also tested like a malignant tumor with color Doppler flow.

Although almost all reports of transvaginal color Doppler ultrasound are enthusiastic regarding the differentiation of benign versus malignant ovarian neoplasms, a recent report from Shimane University in Japan suggested that it does not provide more useful diagnostic information than morphology TVS, magnetic resonance imaging, and serum Ca 125 tests.[105] There was a significant difference between the RI value (0.692 ± 0.188) in benign tumors and in malignant tumors (0.503 ± 0.107). An RI cutoff value of 0.72 was used, which was the mean of the malignant RI + 2 standard deviations. There was considerable overlap of benign and malignant RI, which 25 of the 27 malignancies and 17 of the 36 benign tumors having an RI of less than 0.72. There was no significant difference of RI in relation to stage. The sensitivity and specificity of the RI were 92.6 and 52.8%, respectively. This was not a significant difference from transvaginal ultrasound morphology, with values 85.2 and 69.4%. The RI sensitivity was higher than that of MRI (66.7%) and Ca 125 (59.3%); however, the RI specificity was lower than the MRI (97.1%) and Ca 125 (91.7%).

The authors attributed the overlap to "the advanced instrument with increased Doppler sensitivity (which) allows detection of peripheral parenchymal blood flow signals with low pulsatility in both benign and malignant ovarian tumors."[105] They used the lowest RI of signals from intratumoral and/or tumor surface arteries.

Personal speculation of the previous study is that perhaps surface vessels are stretched or have unilateral compression, thereby reducing the muscle wall resistance. The authors did not mention it, but only 28 of the 63 Japanese women referred for an ovarian mass were postmenopausal, and this might have affected the results. Could it be that Japanese women are thinner, thereby allowing closer proximity to the transducer, or that their vessels are less sclerotic? Clearly, there is a need for an international conference on transvaginal Doppler ultrasound to standardize the equipment and technology to differentiate benign from malignant ovarian neoplasms, and to pool large numbers of cases! Manufacturers have different automatic computer cutoff points of velocity below which no waveform is generated.

There is an inherent difficulty in screening a premenopausal population. In a group of 327 women screened by Harvard Medical School because of family history (one first- or multiple second-degree relatives) of whom 80% were premenopausal, an initial ultrasound examination was abnormal in 51 women (16%), 90% of whom were premenopausal.[106] Because of persistence, laparotomy was done in 10 women and showed 5 benign neoplasms and 5 benign functional cysts. Preoperative Doppler waveforms were obtained in only 6 patients and showed an ominous mean PI of 0.88. The serum Ca 125 level was elevated at more than 35 U/ml in 13%, with a range of 36 to 177 U/ml. All the patients but one were premenopausal, and subsequently half of the cases with elevated Ca 125 serum levels returned to normal levels. The mean serum Ca 125 level was higher and more variable in premenopausal (20 ± 17 U/ml versus postmenopausal (10 ± 6 U/ml) women. One woman had a hysterectomy and bilateral salpingo-oophorectomy for a rising Ca 125 level and was found to have only adenomyosis. Among 12 women who had a prophylactic oophorectomy, no consistent abnormality was found.

While helpful and despite the theoretical aspects, color Doppler sonography is not always 100% reliable in differentiating benign versus malignant ovarian masses.[40] Misdiagnosis may occur in benign inflammatory masses, metabolically active benign neoplasms, and corpus luteum cysts because of their increased and abnormal vascularization.[40]

Clinical study of tumor blood flow (quality, location, type) by transvaginal color Doppler ultrasound may give pathologists an incentive to further investigate blood vessels, perhaps by special endothelial and angiogenesis factor stains or vessel injection. This may give information regarding the change from benign to malignant neoplasia and the prognosis, especially since there is an ultrasound suggestion that neovascularity in cancer precedes obvious gross morphologic change.

It would also be of interest if it could be determined whether neovascularity precedes, is in step with, or follows neoplasm growth.

Perhaps, a biochemical variety of malignant tumors develop. Only those that happen to produce an angiogenesis induction chemical might be able to grow rapidly. Those that did not would remain small and/or be destroyed by the body's immune defenses. In nature, parasites generally do not kill the host and there is evolutionary preselection from host to host. Malignant tumors are fatal, so that there is no evolutionary preselection, and therefore there might be an innumerable variety of tumors.

## PLATES

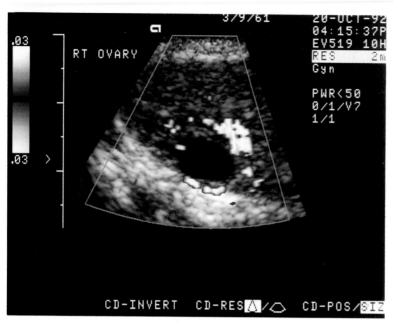

A

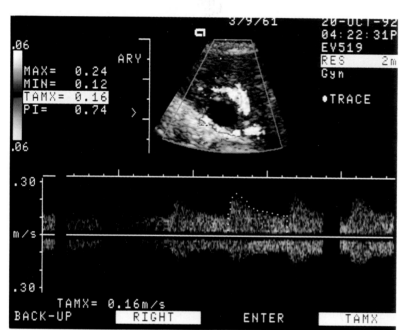

B

**Plate 1-1** Corpus luteum cyst. (A) Transvaginal ultrasound color flow. (B) Transvaginal ultrasound color flow and Doppler waveform. The high diastolic flow (PI 0.74) is similar to that of malignant neovascularity. Therefore in menstruating women, ultrasonography should be done in the proliferative phase to avoid the corpus luteum with its suggestion of malignancy due to the PI's being less than 1. From Dr. Clement M. Barone, New York City.

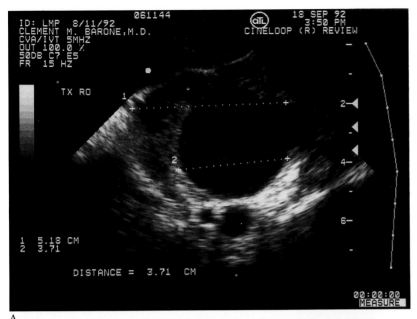

A

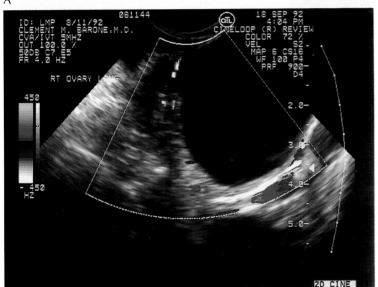

B

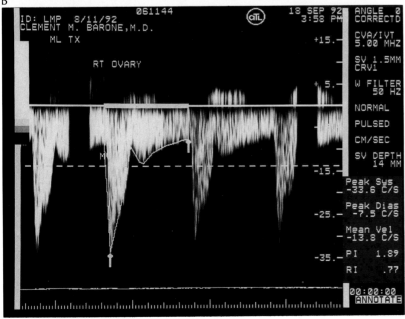

C

**Plate 1-2** (A) Right ovarian cyst, 3.8 cm. Transvaginal ultrasound. (B) Color flow, transvaginal ultrasound. (C) Doppler waveform, transvaginal ultrasound, indicating benign flow with PI 1.89 and RI 0.77. From Dr. Clement M. Barone, New York City.

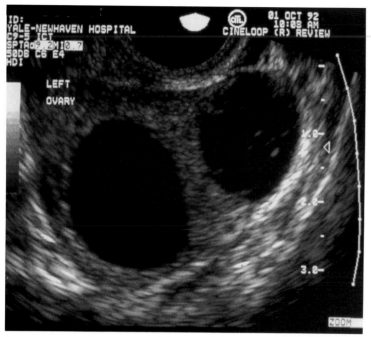

A

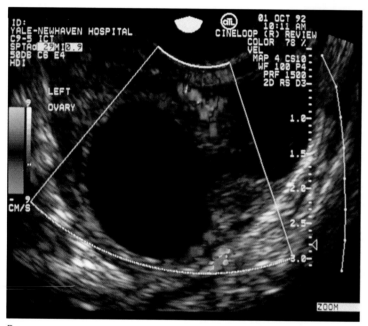

B

**Plate 1-3** Ovarian cyst with thick septum or double cyst.
(A) Transvaginal ultrasound. (B) Color flow transvaginal ultrasound.

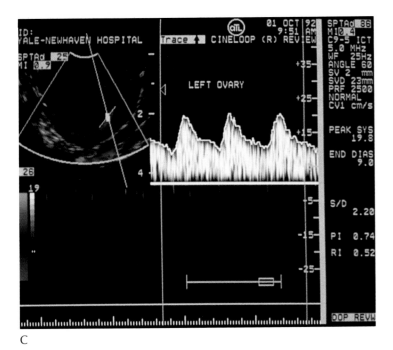

C

**Plate 1-3** (C) Doppler flow wave analysis indicates benign
flow with high diastolic pressure. From Advanced
Technology Lab.

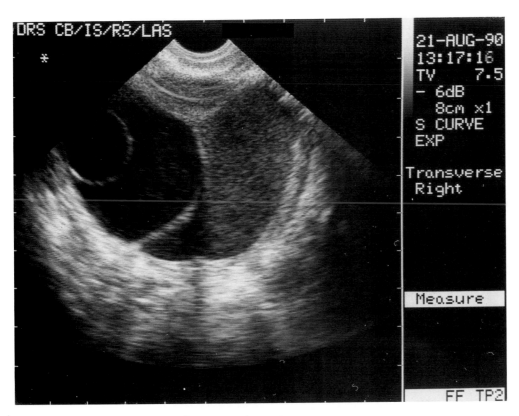

**Plate 1-4** Benign mucinous cystadenoma. Right ovarian complex, cystic multiloculated mass filled with low-level echoes
due to mucin, at surgery was found to be a mucinous cystadenoma. Transvaginal ultrasound. Serous cystadenoma are
similar but usually lack internal echoes. From Drs. Lyris Ann
Schonholz and Claude Bloch, New York City.

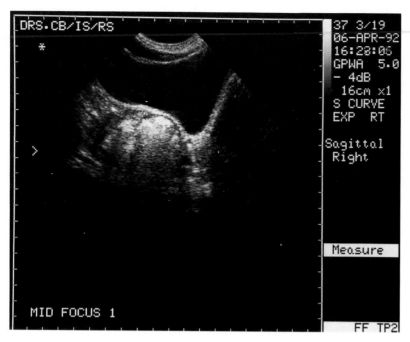

**Plate 1-5** Dermoid cyst (mature cystic teratoma). Right ovarian complex echogenic mass with attenuation. Transabdominal ultrasound. From Drs. Lyris Ann Schonholz and Claude Bloch, New York City.

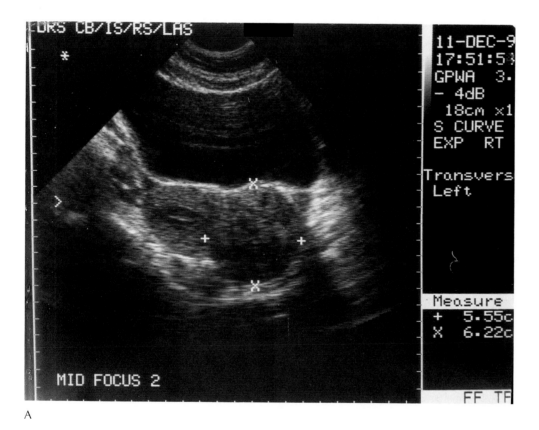

A

**Plate 1-6** Left ovarian thecoma. (A) Solid tumor similar to leiomyoma. From Drs. Lyris Ann Schonholz and Claude Bloch, New York City.

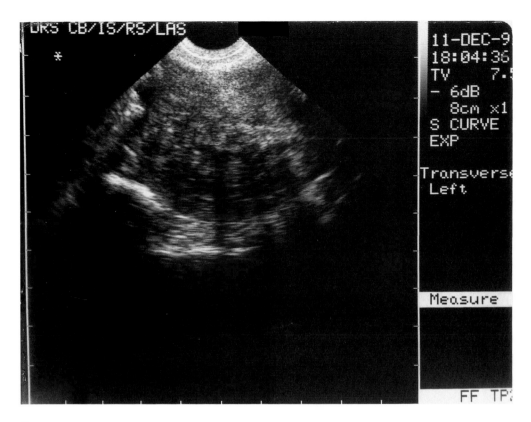

B

**Plate 1-6** (B) Transvaginal ultrasound. From Drs. Lyris Ann
Schonholz and Claude Bloch, New York City.

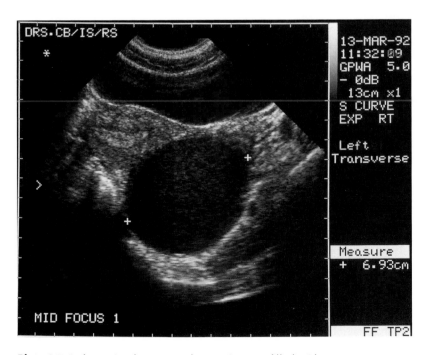

**Plate 1-7** Left ovarian large complex cystic mass filled with
internal low-level echoes due to blood, found to be an endometrioma. From Drs. Lyris Ann Schonholz and Claude
Bloch, New York City.

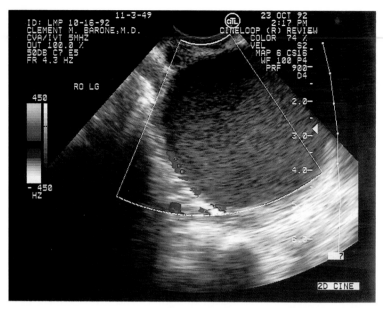

A

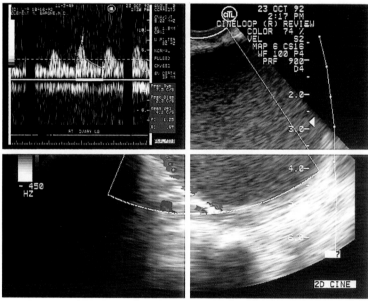

B

**Plate 1-8** Endometrioma of ovary. (A) Transvaginal ultrasound with color flow. (B) Transvaginal ultrasound with color flow and Doppler waveform showing a benign low diastolic flow of PI 1.25 and RI 0.57. From Dr. Clement M. Barone, New York City.

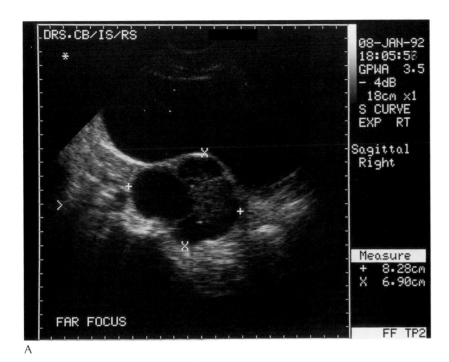

A

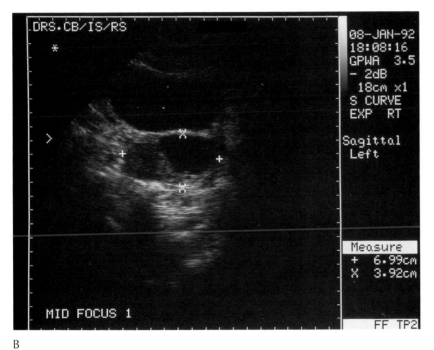

B

**Plate 1-9** Bilateral complex ovarian masses with cystic and solid components due to ovarian cancer, transabdominal ultrasound. (A) Right ovarian mass. (B) Left ovarian mass. From Drs. Lyris Ann Schonholz and Claude Bloch, New York City.

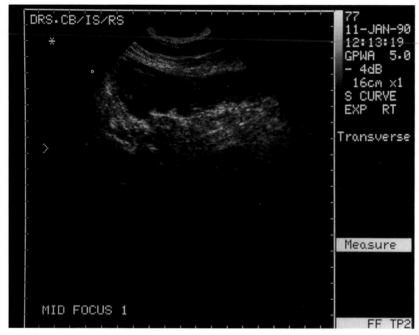

A

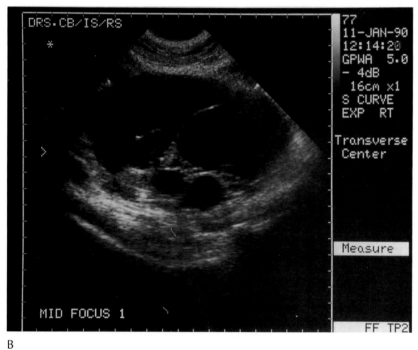

B

**Plate 1-10**  (A) Infiltration of omentum (omental cake) due to
ovarian carcinoma. (B) Large complex multinucleated cystic
ovarian masses with solid components due to ovarian carcinoma. Transabdominal ultrasound. From Drs. Lyris Ann
Schonholz and Claude Bloch, New York City.

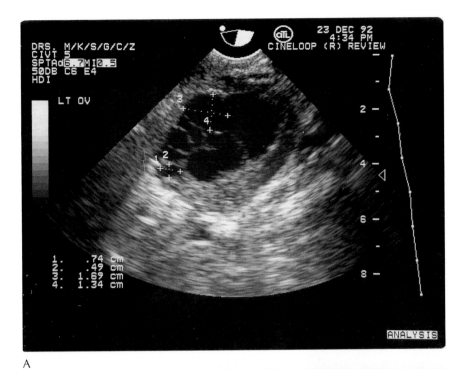

A

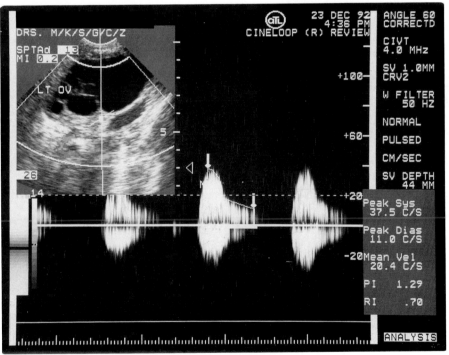

B

**Plate 1-11** (A,B) Bilateral ovarian dominant and smaller cysts with multiple polypoid excrescences, septations, and solid portions suggesting the possibility of malignancy. The Doppler PIs were 1.86 and 1.29, and the RIs were 0.8 and 0.79, which indicated high diastolic pressure and low diastolic flow. Despite these benign flow studies, laparotomy revealed bilateral cystadenocarcinoma. From Drs. D. Maklansky, H. B. Grunther, J. D. Kurzban, R. M. Stoll, B. A. Cohen, J. Zimmer, and A. D. Hyman, New York City.

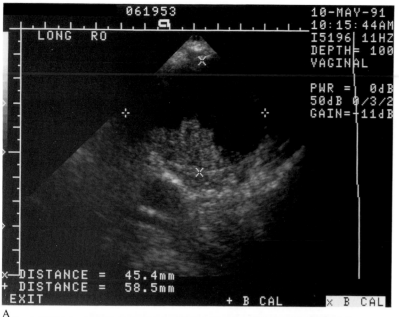

A

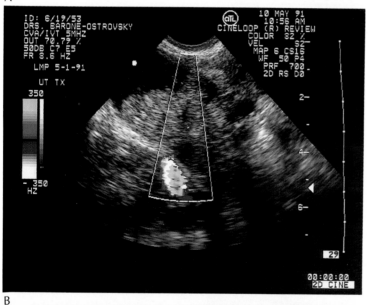

B

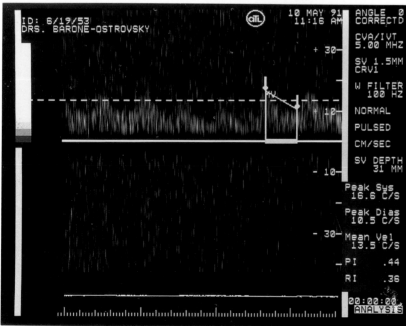

C

**Plate 1-12** Complex right ovarian enlargement with mural nodularity. (A) Transvaginal ultrasound. (B) Color flow. (C) Doppler waveform with PI of 0.44 (suspicious of malignancy if less than 1.00) and RI of 0.36 indicative of high diastolic flow and low diastolic pressure suggestive of malignancy. At laparotomy, an ovarian serous cystadenoma was found with a focus of malignancy. From Dr. Clement M. Barone, New York City.

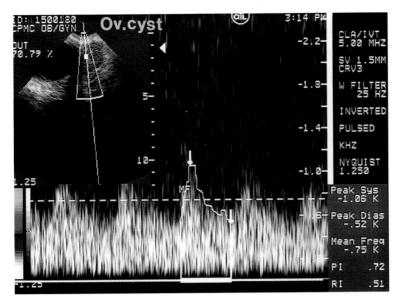

**Plate 1-13** A thin-walled, smooth, sonolucent unilocular left ovarian cyst was subjected to color Doppler flow measurements. The PI was 0.72 and the RI was 0.51. These values are indicative of normal resistance-to-flow values usually seen in benign ovarian masses. The histologic examination confirmed a simple epithelial cyst. From Dr. Ilan Timor-Tritsch, Director of Ob-Gyn Ultrasound, Co-Director of Obstetrical Service, Department of Obstetrics and Gynecology, Columbia University, College of Physicians and Surgeons, New York, New York.

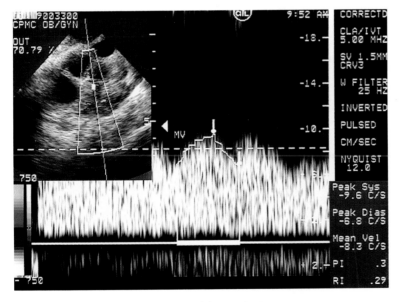

**Plate 1-14** A 6.2 × 5.1 × 4.3 cm right ovarian mass showed thick walls, multiple septa, several high echogenic foci, and internal papillations. The color Doppler–directed resistance-to-flow measurements resulted in a PI of 0.3 and an RI of 0.29, which were indicative of a low-resistance vascular system. The histologic examination of the specimen revealed a well-differentiated adenocarcinoma of the ovary. From Dr. Ilan Timor-Tritsch, Director of Ob-Gyn Ultrasound, Co-Director of Obstetrical Service, Department of Obstetrics and Gynecology, Columbia University, College of Physicians and Surgeons, New York, New York.

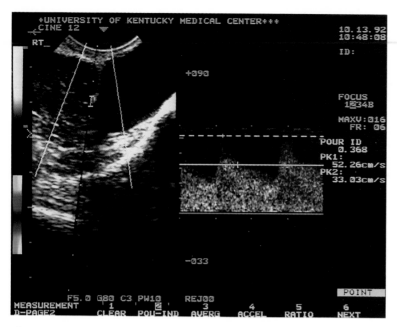

**Plate 1-15** Doppler flow sonogram of cystic ovarian tumor (volume at 25.3 cm³) with blood flow having a normal (>4.0) RI of 0.794. From Dr. J. R. van Nagell Jr., Director Gynecologic Oncology, University of Kentucky, Lexington, Kentucky.

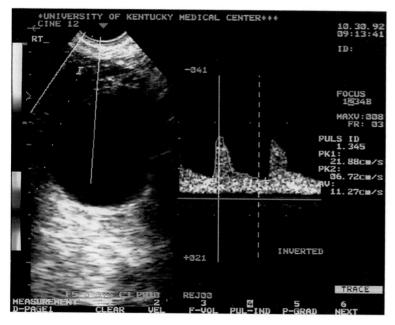

**Plate 1-16** Doppler flow sonogram of cystic ovarian tumor (volume 52.2 cm³) with blood flow having an abnormal (<0.4) RI of 0.368. From Dr. J. R. van Nagell Jr., Director Gynecologic Oncology, University of Kentucky, Lexington, Kentucky.

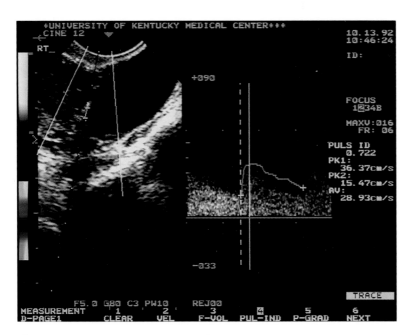

**Plate 1-17** Doppler flow sonogram of cystic ovarian tumor (volume 21.9 cm³) with blood flow having a normal (1.0) PI of 1.345. From Dr. J. R. van Nagell Jr., Director Gynecologic Oncology, University of Kentucky, Lexington, Kentucky.

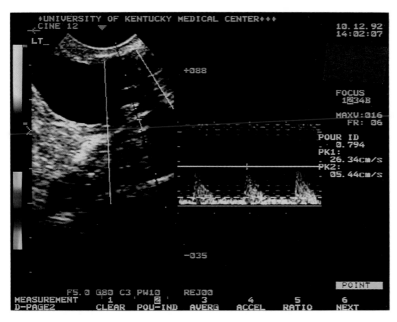

**Plate 1-18** Doppler flow sonogram of cystic ovarian tumor (volume 35.4 cm³) with blood flow having an abnormal (<1.0) pulsatility index of 0.722. From Dr. J. R. van Nagell Jr., Director Gynecologic Oncology, University of Kentucky, Lexington, Kentucky.

## REFERENCES

1. Boring CC, Squires TS, Tong T. Cancer statistics, 1993. *CA* 43:7–26, 1993.
2. *Cancer Facts Figures—1992.* Atlanta, American Cancer Society, 1992.
3. Ozols RF. Ovarian cancer, Part II: Treatment. In *Current Problems in Cancer,* vol. 16, no. 2 (March/April). New York, Mosby Year Book, 1992, p 69 (3A), p 72 (3B).
4. Townsend J. *Strengthening Research in Academic Ob/Gyn Departments.* Washington, DC, National Academy Press, 1992, pp 195–197.
5. Partridge EE, Gunter BC, Gelder MS, et al. The validity and significance of substages of advanced ovarian cancer. *Gynecol Oncol* 48:236–241, 1993.
6. Parazzini F, Franceschi S, LaVecchia C, Fasoli M. Review: The epidemiology of ovarian cancer. *Gynecol Oncol* 43:9–23, 1991.
7. Harlap S. The epidemiology of ovarian cancer. In *Cancer of the Ovary,* Markman M, Hoskins WJ, eds. New York, Raven, 1993, pp 79–93.
8. Curtin JP. Diagnosis and staging of epithelial ovarian cancer. In *Cancer of the Ovary,* Markman M, Hoskins WJ, eds. New York, Raven, 1993, pp 153–162.
9. Piver MS, Baker TR, Piedmonte M, San Decki, AM. Epidemiology and etiology of ovarian cancer. *Semin Oncol* 18:177–185, 1991.
10. Goldberg GL, Runowicz CD. Ovarian carcinoma of low malignant potential, infertility and induction of ovulation—Is there a link? *Am J Obstet Gynecol* 166:853–854, 1992.
11. Whittemore AS, Harris R, Itnyre J, et al. Characteristics relating to ovarian cancer risk: Collaborative analysis of 12 US case control studies: II. Invasive epithelial cancers in white women. *Am J Epidemiol* 136:1184–1203, 1992.
12. Harris R, Whittemore A, Itnyre J, et al. Characteristics relating to ovarian cancer risk: Collaborative analysis of 12 US case control studies: III. Epithelial tumors of low malignant potential in white women. *Am J Epidemiol* 136:1204–1211, 1992.
13. Whittemore AS, Harris R, Itnyre J, et al. Characteristics relating to ovarian cancer risk: Collaborative analysis of 12 US case control studies: IV. The pathogenesis of epithelial ovarian cancer. *Am J Epidemiol* 136:1212–1220, 1992.
14. Parazzini F, Negri E, LaVecchia C, Luchini L, Mezzopane R. Hysterectomy oophorectomy and subsequent ovarian cancer risk. *Obstet Gynecol* 81:363–366, 1993.
15. Hankinson SE, Colditz GA, Hunter DJ, Spencer TL, Rosner B, Stampfer MS. A quantitative assessment of oral contraceptive use and risk of ovarian cancer. *Obstet Gynecol* 80:708–714, 1992.
16. Emons G, Ortmann O, Pahwa GS, Hackenberg R, Oberheuser F, Schulz K-D. Intracellular actions of gonadotropic and peptide hormones and the therapeutic value of GnRH-agonists in ovarian cancer. *Acta Obstet Gynecol Scand* 71(suppl 155):31–38, 1992.
17. Trimble EL, Karlan BY, Lagasse LD, Hoskins WJ. Diagnosing the correct ovarian cancer syndrome. *Obstet Gynecol* 78:1023–1026, 1991.
18. Lynch HT, Lynch JF, Conway TA. Hereditary ovarian cancer. In *Ovarian Cancer,* Rubin SC, Sutton GP, eds. New York, McGraw-Hill, 1993, pp 189–217.
19. Hoskins IA, Ostrer H. Hereditary/familial ovarian cancer. In *Cancer of the Ovary,* Markman M, Hoskins WJ, eds. New York, Raven, 1993, pp 95–113.
20. Piver MS, Recio FO. When is ovarian cancer screening helpful? *Contemporary Ob/Gyn* 38(2):17–18, 21–22, 27–28, 30, 32, 1993.
21. Lynch HT. Genetic risk in ovarian cancer (editorial). *Gynecol Oncol* 46:1–3, 1992.
22. Lynch HT, Cavilieri RJ, Lynch JF, Casey MJ. Case report: Gynecologic cancer clues to Lynch syndrome II diagnosis: A family report. *Gynecol Oncol* 44:198–203, 1992.
23. Blanchet-Bardon C, Nazzaro V, Chverant-Breton J, Espie M, Kerbrat D, LeMarec B. Hereditary epidermolytic palmoplantar keratoderma associated with breast and ovarian cancer in a large kindred. *Br J Dermatol* 117:363–370, 1987.
24. Amos CI, Shaw GL, Tucker MA, Hartge P. Age at onset for familial epithelial ovarian cancer. *JAMA* 268:1896–1899, 1992.
25. Kemp GM, Hsiu J-G, Andrews MC. Case report: Papillary peritoneal carcinomatosis after prophylactic oophorectomy. *Gynecol Oncol* 47:395–397, 1992.
26. Raju U, Fine G, Greenawald KA, Ohorodnik JM. Primary papillary serous neoplasia of the peritoneum: A clinicopathologic and ultrastructural study of eight cases. *Hum Pathol* 20:426–436, 1989.
27. Ryuko K, Miura H, Abu-Musa A, Iwanari O, Kitao M. Case Report: Endosalpingiosis in association with ovarian surface papillary tumor or borderline malignancy. *Gynecol Oncol* 46:107–110, 1992.
28. Shiraki M, Otis CN, Donovan JT, Powell JL. Case Report: Ovarian serous borderline epithelial tumors with multiple retroperitoneal nodal involvement: Metastasis or malignant transformation of epithelial glandular inclusions? *Gynecol Oncol* 46:255–258, 1992.
29. Kerlikowske K, Brown JS, Grady DG. Reviews: Should women with familial ovarian cancer undergo prophylactic oophorectomy? *Obstet Gynecol* 80:700–707, 1992.
30. Berchuk A, Bast RC Jr. Oncogenes and tumor-suppressor genes. In *Ovarian Cancer,* Rubin SC, Sulton GP, eds. New York, McGraw-Hill, 1993, pp 21–37, 34.
31. Tropé C, Makar A, Koern J. DNA flow cytometry as a new prognostic factor in ovarian malignancies (review). *Acta Obstet Gynecol Scand* 71(suppl 155):95–98, 1992.
32. Drescher CW, Flint A, Hopkins MP, Roberts JA. Prognostic significance of DNA content and nuclear morphology in borderline ovarian tumors. *Gynecol Oncol* 48:242–246, 1993.
33. Rotmensch J, Atcher RW, Schwartz JL, Grdina DJ. Analysis of ascites from patients with ovarian carcinoma by cell flow cytometry. *Gynecol Oncol* 44:10–12, 1992.
34. Narod SA, Feunteun J, Lynch HT, et al. Familial breast-

ovarian cancer locus on chromosome 17q12-q23. *Lancet* 338:82–83, 1991.

35. Seidman JD, Frisman DM, Norris HJ. Expression of the *HER-w/neu* proto-oncogene in serous ovarian neoplasms. *Cancer* 70:2857–2860, 1992.

36. Børresen A-L. Oncogenesis in ovarian cancer. *Acta Obstet Gynecol Scand* 71(suppl 155):25–30, 1992.

37. Griffin C. Is ovarian cancer a clonal disease? (editorial). *Gynecol Oncol* 48:1–3, 1993.

38. Tsao S-W, Mok C-H, Knapp RC, et al. Molecular genetic evidence of a unifocal origin for human serous ovarian carcinomas. *Gynecol Oncol* 48:5–10, 1993.

39. Young RH, Welch WR, Dickersin GR, Scully RE. Ovarian sex cord tumor with annular tubules: Review of 74 cases including 27 with Peutz-Jeghers syndrome and four with adenoma malignum of the cervix. *Cancer* 50:1384–1402, 1982.

40. Podczaski E, Kaminski PF, Pees RC, Singapuri K, Sorosky JI. Peutz-Jeghers syndrome with ovarian sex cord tumor with annular tubules and cervical adenoma malignum. *Gynecol Oncol* 42:74–78, 1991.

41. Tanaka Y, Sasaki Y, Nishihira H. Ovarian juvenile granulosa cell tumor associated with Maffucci's syndrome. *Am J Clin Pathol* 97:523–527, 1992.

42. Tamimi HK, Bolen JW. Enchondromatosis (Ollier's disease) and ovarian juvenile granulosa cell tumor. *Cancer* 53:1605–1608, 1984.

43. Weyl-Ben-Arush M, Oslander L. Ollier's disease with ovarian Sertoli-Leydig cell tumor and breast adenoma. *Am J Pediatr Hematol Oncol* 13:49–51, 1991.

44. Pounder DJ, Iyer PV, Davy ML. Bilateral juvenile granulosa cell tumours associated with skeletal enchondromas. *Aust NZ J Obstet Gynaecol* 25(2):123–126, 1985.

45. Khalid BA, Bond AG, Ennis G, Medley G. Dysgerminoma-gonadoblastoma and familial 46XY pure gonadal dysgenesis: Case report and review of the genetics and pathophysiology of gonadal dysgenesis and H-Y antigen. *Aust NZ J Obstet Gynaecol* 22:175–179, 1982.

46. Sinisi AA, Perrone L, Quarto C, Barone M, Bellastella A, Faggiano M. Dysgerminoma in 45X Turner syndrome: Report of a case. *Clin Endocrinol* 28:187–193, 1988.

47. Navot D, Williams MC. The uterus without ovaries. In *The Uterus*, Altchek A, Deligdisch L, eds. New York, Springer-Verlag, 1991, pp 294–299.

48. Barber HRK. *Ovarian Carcinoma. Etiology, Diagnosis, and Treatment*, 3d ed. New York, Springer-Verlag, 1993, p 90.

49. Barber HRK. Epithelial Ovarian Cancer. In *Clinical Gynecologic Oncology*, 4th ed, DiSaia PJ, Creasman WT, eds. St. Louis, Mosby Year Book, 1993, pp 333–425.

50. Morrow CP. Malignant and borderline epithelial tumors of ovary: Clinical features, staging, diagnosis, intraoperative assessment and review of management. In *Gynecologic Oncology, Fundamental Principles and Clinical Practice*, 2d ed, Coppleson M, Monaghan JM, Morrow CP, Tattersall MHN, eds. New York, Churchill Livingstone, 1992, p 892 (50A), p 893 (50B).

51. Carter J, Carson LF, Byers L, et al. Transvaginal ultra-sound in gynecologic oncology (review). *Obstet Gynecol Surv* 46:687–696, 1991.

52. Piver MS, Fanning J, Craig KA. Ovarian cancer. *Gynecologic Oncology*, 2d ed, Knapp RC, Berkowitz RS, eds. New York, McGraw-Hill, 1993, p 254.

53. Jacobs IJ, Oram DH, Bast RC Jr. Strategies for improving the specificity of screening for ovarian cancer with tumor-associated antigens Ca 125, Ca 15-3, and TAG 72.3. *Obstet Gynecol* 80:396–399, 1992.

54. Bourne TH, Whitehead ML, Campbell S, et al. Ultrasound screening for familial ovarian cancer. *Gynecol Oncol* 43:92–97, 1991.

55. Berchuck A, Boente MP, Bast RC Jr. The use of tumor markers in the management of patients with gynecologic carcinomas. *Clin Obstet Gynecol* 35:45–54, 1992.

56. Jacobs I, Bast RC Jr. Clinical review: The Ca 125 tumour-associated antigen: A review of the literature. *Hum Reprod* 4:1–12, 1989.

57. Welander CE. What do Ca 125 and other antigens tell us about ovarian cancer biology? *Acta Obstet Gynecol Scand* 71(suppl 155):85–93, 1992.

58. Grover S, Koh H, Weideman P, Quinn MA, et al. The effect of the menstrual cycle on serum Ca 125 levels: A population study. *Am J Obstet Gynecol* 167:1379–1381, 1992.

59. O'Shaughnessy A, Check JH, Nowroozi K, et al. Ca 125 levels measured in different phases of the menstrual cycle in screening for endometriosis. *Obstet Gynecol* 81:99–103, 1993.

60. Williams LL, Fleischer AC, Jones HW III. Case report: Transvaginal color Doppler sonography and Ca 125 elevation in a patient with ovarian thecoma and ascites. *Gynecol Oncol* 46:115–118, 1992.

61. Negishi Y, Iwabuchi H, Sakunaga H, et al. Serum and tissue measurements of CA 72-4 in ovarian cancer patients. *Gynecol Oncol* 48:148–154, 1993.

62. Gadducci A, Ferdeghini M, Prontera C, et al. The concomitant determination of different tumor markers in patients with epithelial ovarian cancer and benign ovarian masses: Relevance for differential diagnosis. *Gynecol Oncol* 44:147–154, 1992.

63. Devine PL, McGuckin MA, Ward BG. Circulating mucins as tumor markers in ovarian cancer (review). *Anticancer Res* 3:709–717, 1992.

64. van-Niekerk CC, Boerman OC, Ramaekers FC, Poels LG. Marker profile of different phases in the transition of normal human ovarian epithelium to ovarian carcinomas. *Am J Pathol* 138:455–463, 1991.

65. Rice LW, Lage JM, Berkowitz RS, et al. Preoperative serum Ca 125 levels in borderline tumors of the ovary. *Gynecol Oncol* 46:226–229, 1992.

66. Hunter VJ, Weinberg JB, Haney AF, et al. Ca 125 in peritoneal fluid and serum from patients with benign gynecologic conditions and ovarian cancer. *Gynecol Oncol* 36:161–165, 1990.

67. Vergote IB, Onsrud M, Børmer OP. Ca 125 in peritoneal fluid of ovarian cancer patients. *Gynecol Oncol* 44:161–165, 1992.

68. Makar APH, Tropé CG. Endometrial and ovarian ma-

lignancies: Epidemiology, etiology and prognostic factors. *Acta Obstet Gynecol Scand* 71:331–336, 1992.

69. Sevelda P, Rosen A, Denison U, et al. Is Ca-125 monitoring useful in patients with epithelial ovarian carcinoma and preoperative negative Ca 125 serum levels? *Gynecol Oncol* 43:154–158, 1991.

70. Mogensen O. Prognostic value of Ca 125 in advanced ovarian cancer. *Gynecol Oncol* 44:207–212, 1992.

71. Hosono MN, Endo K, Sakahara H. Different antigenic nature in apparently healthy women with high serum Ca 125 levels compared with typical patients with ovarian cancer. *Cancer* 70:2851–2856, 1992.

72. van Nagell JR Jr, DePriest PD. Early diagnosis of epithelial ovarian cancer. In *Cancer of the Ovary*, Markman M, Hoskins WJ, eds. New York, Raven, 1993, p 128.

73. Campbell S, Bhan V, Royston P, Whitehead MI, Collins WP. Transabdominal ultrasound screening for early ovarian cancer. *Br Med J* 299:1363–1367, 1989.

74. Campbell S, Royston P, Bhan V, Whitehead MI, Collins WP. Novel screening strategies for early ovarian cancer by transabdominal ultrasonography. *Br J Obstet Gynecol* 97:304–311, 1990.

75. Andolf E, Svalenius E, Astedt B. Ultrasonography for early detection of ovarian carcinoma. *J Obstet Gynaecol* 93:1286–1289, 1976.

76. Jones HW III. Commentary. *Obstet Gynecol Surv* 47:55, 1992.

77. van Nagell JR Jr, DePriest PD, Puls LE, et al. Ovarian cancer screening in asymptomic postmenopausal women by transvaginal sonography. *Cancer* 68:458–462, 1991.

78. Wolf SI, Gosink BB, Feldesman MR, et al. Prevalence of simple adnexal cysts in postmenopausal women. *Radiology* 180:65–71, 1991.

79. Jacobs I, Stabile I, Bridges J, et al. Multimodal approach to screening for ovarian cancer. *Lancet* 1:268–271, 1988.

80. Granberg S, Wikland M. Endovaginal ultrasound in the diagnosis of unilocular ovarian cysts in postmenopausal women. *Ultrasound Q* 10:1–13, 1992.

81. Sassone AM, Timor-Tritsch IE, Artner A, Westhoff C, Warren WB. Transvaginal sonographic characterization of ovarian disease: Evaluation of a new scoring system to predict ovarian malignancy. *Obstet Gynecol* 78:70–76, 1991.

82. Granberg S, Wikland M, Jansson I. Macroscopic characterization of ovarian tumors and the relation to the histological diagnosis: Criteria to be used for ultrasound evaluation. *Gynecol Oncol* 35:139–144, 1989.

83. Benacerraf BR, Finkler NJ, Wojciechowski C, Knapp RC. Sonographic accuracy in the diagnosis of ovarian masses. *J Reprod Med* 35:491–495, 1990.

84. DePriest PD, Shenson A, Fried J, et al. A morphology index based on sonographic findings in ovarian tumors. 24th Annual Meeting of the Society of Gynecologic Oncologists, February 7–10, Palm Desert, California. Abstract 59 *Gyn Oncol* 49:122, 1993.

85. Hata K, Hata T, Makihara K, et al. Preoperative diagnostic imaging of normal-sized ovary carcinoma syndrome. *Int J Gynaecol Obstet* 35:259–264, 1991.

86. Levine D, Gosink BB, Wolf SI, et al. Simple adnexal cysts: The natural history of postmenopausal women. *Radiology* 184:653–659, 1992.

87. Bret PM, Atri M. Guibaud L, et al. Ovarian cysts in postmenopausal women: Preliminary results with transvaginal alcohol sclerosis. Work in progress. *Radiology* 184:661–663, 1992.

88. Kurjak A, Schulman H, Sosic A, Zalud I, Shalan H. Transvaginal ultrasound, color flow and Doppler waveform of the postmenopausal adnexal mass. *Obstet Gynecol* 80:917–921.

89. Nezhat F, Nezhat C, Welander CE, Benigno B. Four ovarian cancers diagnosed during laparoscopic management of 1011 women with adnexal masses. *Am J Obstet Gynecol* 167:790–796, 1992.

90. Dershaw DD, Panicek DM. Radiologic evaluation of ovarian cancer. In *Cancer of the Ovary*, Markman M, Hoskins WJ, eds. New York, Raven, 1993, pp 133–152.

91. Kurjak A, Zalud I. Ultrasound assessment of adnexal masses. In *Color Doppler Imaging in Obstetrics and Gynecology*, Jaffe R, Warsof SL, eds. New York, McGraw-Hill, 1992, pp 265–282.

92. Kurjak A, Zalud I, Jurkovic D, Alfirević Ž, Miljan M. Transvaginal color Doppler for the assessment of pelvic circulation. *Acta Obstet Gynecol Scand* 68:131–135, 1989.

93. Bourne T, Campbell S, Steer C, Whitehead MI, Collins WP. Transvaginal colour flow imaging: A possible new screening technique for ovarian cancer. *Br Med J* 299: 1367–1370, 1989.

94. Folkman J, Watson K, Ingber D, Folkman J. Induction of angiogenesis during the transition from hyperplasia to neoplasia. *Nature* 339:58–61, 1989.

95. Kurjak A, Žalud I: Tumor neovascularization. In *Transvaginal Color Doppler, A Comprehensive Guide to Transvaginal Color Doppler Sonography in Obstetrics and Gynecology*, Kurjak A, ed. Park Ridge, New Jersey, Parthenon Publishing Group, pp 93–101.

96. Fleischer AC, Rodgers WH, Kepple DM, et al. Color Doppler sonography of benign and malignant ovarian masses. *Radiographics* 12:879–885, 1992.

97. Kremkau FW. Principles and instrumentation. In *Doppler Color Imaging*, Merritt CRB, ed. New York, Churchill Livingstone, 1992, pp 7–60.

98. Meyer WJ, Jaffe R. Basic principles of Doppler ultrasonography. In *Color Doppler Imaging in Obstetrics and Gynecology*, Jaffe R, Warsof SL, eds. New York, McGraw-Hill, 1992, pp 1–16.

99. Kawai M, Kano T, Kikkawa F, Maeda O, Oguchi H, Tomoda Y. Transvaginal Doppler ultrasound with color flow imaging in the diagnosis of ovarian cancer. *Obstet Gynecol* 79:163–167, 1992.

100. Timor-Tritsch IE, Lerner JP, Monteagudo A, Santos R. Transvaginal sonographic characterization of ovarian masses using color flow directed Doppler measurements and a morphologic scoring system. *Am J Obstet Gynecol* 168:909–913, 1993.

101. Weiner Z, Thaler I, Beck D, Rottem S, Deutsch M, Brandes JM. Differentiating malignant from benign ovarian tumors with transvaginal color flow imaging. *Obstet Gynecol* 79:159–162, 1992.

102. Kurjak A, Salihagic A, Kupesic-Urek S, Predanic A. Review article: Clinical value of the assessment of gynaecological tumour angiogenesis by transvaginal colour doppler. *Ann Med* 24:97–103, 1992.

103. Kurjak A, Predanić M. New scoring system for prediction of ovarian malignancy based on transvaginal color Doppler sonography. *J Ultrasound Med* 11:631–638, 1992.

104. Hata K, Hata T, Manabe A, Kitao M. Ovarian tumors of low malignant potential: Transvaginal Doppler ultrasound features. *Gynecol Oncol* 45:259–264, 1992.

105. Hata K, Hata T, Manabe A, Sugimura K, Kitao M. A critical evaluation of transvaginal Doppler studies, transvaginal sonography, magnetic resonance imaging and Ca 125 in detecting ovarian cancer. *Obstet Gynecol* 80:922–926, 1992.

106. Muto MG, Cramer DW, Brown DL, et al. Screening for ovarian cancer: The preliminary experience of a familial ovarian cancer center. 24th Annual Meeting of the Gynecologic Oncologists, February 7–10, 1993, Palm Desert, California. Abstract 20 *Gyn Oncol* 49, p 112, 1993.

## RECOMMENDED GENERAL REFERENCES

Barber HRK. *Ovarian Carcinoma. Etiology, Diagnosis and Treatment*, 3d ed. New York, Springer-Verlag, 1993.

Coppleson M, Monaghan JM, Morrow CP, Tattersall MHN, eds. *Gynecologic Oncology, Fundamental Principles and Clinical Practice*, 2d ed. New York, Churchill Livingstone, 1992, vols 1 and 2.

DiSaia PJ, Creasman WT. *Clinical Gynecologic Oncology*, 4th ed. St. Louis, Mosby Year Book, 1993.

Greer BE, Berek JS. *Gynecologic Oncology Treatment Rationale and Techniques*. New York, Elsevier, 1991.

Hamilton TC. Ovarian cancer: I. Biology, vol 16, no 1. *Curr Probl Cancer* 16:1–57, 1992.

Hoskins WJ, Perez CA, Young RC, eds. *Principles and Practice of Gynecologic Oncology*. Philadelphia, Lippincott, 1992.

Jaffe R, Warsof SL. *Color Doppler Imaging in Obstetrics and Gynecology*. New York, McGraw-Hill, 1992.

Knapp RC, Berkowitz RS, eds. *Gynecologic Oncology*, 2d ed. New York, McGraw-Hill, 1993.

Kurjak A, ed. *Transvaginal Color Doppler. A Comprehensive Guide to Transvaginal Color Doppler Sonography in Obstetrics and Gynecology*. Park Ridge, New Jersey, Parthenon Publishing Group, 1991.

Markman M, Hoskins WJ eds. *Cancer of the Ovary*. New York, Raven, 1993.

Merritt CRB, ed. *Doppler Color Imaging*. New York, Churchill Livingstone, 1992.

Ozols RF, guest ed. *Ovarian cancer, Seminars in Oncology*. Saunders Harcourt Brace Jovanovich, 1991, 18(3).

Ozols RF. *Ovarian cancers: II. Treatment. Curr Probl Cancer* 16(2):61–126, 1992.

Rubin SC, Sutton GP, ed. *Ovarian Cancer*. New York, McGraw-Hill, 1993.

Runowicz CD. Advances in the screening and treatment of ovarian cancer. *CA* 42(6):327–349, 1992.

Sutton CL, McKinney CD, Jones JE, Gay SB. Ovarian masses revisited: Radiologic and pathologic correlation. *Radiographics* 12:853–877, 1992.

Timor-Tritsch IE, Rottem S, eds. *Transvaginal Sonography*, 2nd ed. New York, Elsevier, 1991.

# 2

# Management of Malignant Epithelial Tumors of the Ovary

*Carmel J. Cohen, M.D.*

Malignant neoplasms of the ovary present the gynecologic oncologist with the most challenging problems in screening, detection, therapy, and prevention because of the ubiquitous nature of these cancers and the imperfect understanding of their development and biology. While ovarian cancer accounts for only 4% of malignant neoplasms occurring in the female, the sixth most common female cancer, there are more annual deaths (13,000) in the United States than there are from the more commonly occurring cancers of the endometrium and cervix combined. The risk of acquiring ovarian cancer after the age of 40 years is approximately 1.6%, and, while there are some groups at slightly higher risk, any woman with an ovary is at risk for the disease.

Because ovarian cancer may metastasize early and because a 1-cm³ enlargement in the ovary represents a volume of $10^9$ epithelial ovarian cancer cells, this disease is detected only after it has spread from the ovary in 70 to 75% of patients with ovarian cancer. Since the cure rate for patients with well-differentiated stage I ovarian cancers (those cancers confined to the ovary with intact capsules and negative cytologic washings) can be as high as 90% by simple surgical removal, the assumption has been made that improved diagnostic techniques will discover a higher percentage of stage I ovary cancers, resulting in improved cure rates.

However, there is indirect evidence that many of the cancers assigned to the ovary may, in fact, be simultaneous expressions of an oncogene on a target with homogeneously derived embryologic origin—the peritoneum. This suggestion derives from the observations that mesothelial surfaces in patients who have ovarian cancer demonstrate disorders of morphometry in areas away from the primary cancer; women have been observed to develop "ovarian cancer" after prophylactic oophorectomy in the cancer-prone families; and there is a large collection of women with widespread "ovarian carcinoma" in whom the ovaries show histologic evidence of carcinoma on the ovarian capsule without the histologic parameters suggesting the ovaries as a primary site. These considerations strengthen the requirement for detection techniques that do not rely on ovarian size alone. An ideal exquisitely sensitive serodiagnostic technique for ovarian cancer has not yet been perfected. For now, a variety of currently available markers along with pelvic examination and noninvasive radiography provide the best opportunity for early diagnosis.

While the ultimate diagnosis of ovarian cancer depends on obtaining tissue for pathologic examination, the presence of an adnexal mass in the postmenopausal state or an enlarging adnexal mass unresponsive to hormonal regulation in the premenopausal state should raise suspicions of ovarian neoplasia. If benignity cannot be established by analysis of radiographic patterns or unchanging size in a period of careful observation, histologic examination is essential. Percutaneous sonographically guided needle biopsy, laparoscopic oophorectomy, or removal of tissue by laparotomy are the techniques conventionally available for histologic diagnosis. Ideally a technique should be chosen that does not permit rupture of a cystic mass or spill of tumor from incomplete removal; this usually translates to exploratory laparotomy. If, however, the mass is cystic, not larger than 6 cm, and not complex, laparoscopic removal of the intact ovary by salpingo-oophorectomy and retrieval of the specimen through a protective plastic bag through which cyst aspiration might be performed, thus allowing removal through a widened laparoscopic port, is acceptable. This method should only be employed by experienced laparoscopists and only in a circumstance in which no spillage occurs and an immediate histologic report is available. Should there be a malignant neoplasm, we recommend immediate laparotomy with full surgical staging and treatment. Percutaneous needle biopsy should be reserved for those patients with metastatic disease who are too ill to tolerate other invasive procedures.

Classically, surgical staging for ovarian carcinoma is performed through a laparotomy approach that permits full access to all quadrants of the peritoneal cavity. In most hands this requires a vertical incision extending from the symphysis, usually midline, and including the epigastrium. There are surgeons who prefer a transverse hypogastric muscle–cutting incision that by virtue of its length and placement allows equal access to the pelvis and to the epigastrium.

Upon entry, any fluid from the peritoneal cavity is collected for cytologic examination. If fluid is not present, then at least 200 ml of saline is instilled, the abdominal contents are thus lavaged, and the saline is retrieved for a cytologic analysis. A careful exploration of the abdomen and the retroperitoneum is essential. Paradoxically the earliest stage requires the most careful and exhaustive staging procedure for verification. If the disease appears grossly confined to one ovary, histologic proof requires sampling the contralateral ovary; removing the omentum; sampling the pelvic and paraaortic lymph nodes; randomly biopsying sites from the lateral colonic gutters and the pelvic walls; and cytologic swabbing or histologic sampling of the anterior parietal peritoneum and/or diaphragms overlying the liver. When this has been done in patients with true stage I disease in whom the ovarian capsule is intact and the tumor is well differentiated, further treatment after the surgery has not been demonstrated to improve cure. In young patients who have been appropriately counseled, who desire further reproduction, and who are willing to submit to close surveillance, there is no evidence that surgery other then wide unilateral salpingo-oophorectomy enhances cure. However, since there may be sequential bilaterality in epithelial ovarian cancer, we

recommended that when childbearing is completed, the uterus and contralateral ovary be removed and restaging be performed.

For postmenopausal patients, for those who have disease more advanced than stage I, or for those with earlier disease who have completed their childbearing, most therapists would recommend an abdominal hysterectomy with bilateral salpingo-oophorectomy, omentectomy, lymph node sampling for early disease, lymphadenectomy in a cytoreductive effort for later disease, and an ultimate attempt to remove all disease consistent with maintaining a physiologic plateau. While there are different views on the role of bowel surgery in this cytoreductive effort, our experience suggests that the removal of all gross disease improves survival. Thus we include a mechanical and antimicrobial bowel preparation for all patients suspected of having ovarian carcinoma and we remove bowel when necessary in order to achieve ideal cytoreduction. It is rarely necessary at the time of initial cytoreduction to perform a colostomy in patients previously untreated even when there is widespread disease on the surfaces of large and small bowel. Ten years ago in our institution, 25% of our patients with stages III and IV ovarian cancer were treated with ideal initial cytoreductive surgery (residual disease less than 2 cm). Today this figure is closer to 50%, a result of improved techniques, better-trained surgical teams, and a strong belief in the utility of maximal surgical cytoreduction prior to adjunctive therapy.

While there is controversy on the role of cytoreduction, with some arguing that less virulent disease lends itself to cytoreduction and thus those patients achieving cytoreduction respond better and live longer, until a prospective study disproves the value of cytoreduction we continue to pursue it because there is virtually no experience among gynecologic oncologists suggesting that patients do better without it. Moreover, experimental experiences with cell cultures, organ cultures, and animals all support the value of cytoreduction prior to cytotoxic nonsurgical therapy in most neoplastic processes. Recently we have treated young patients who have stage III ovarian cancer, who wish to retain reproductive function, and in whom retention of the uterus did not seem to diminish prognosis. In these patients, there is a possibility for primary cytoreduction including bilateral oophorectomy, uterine retention, subsequent treatment with cytotoxic therapy, identification of probability of cure, and exploitation of the retained uterus for in vitro fertilization with ovum donation. We recommend removal of the uterus after childbearing is complete.

Upon completion of the first surgical treatment, the options available for continued treatment for patients with epithelial ovarian cancers include radiation therapy, cytotoxic chemotherapy, hormonal therapy, and active or passive immunotherapy or biologic response modification.

There is evidence that when all gross disease has been removed from patients with epithelial ovarian cancer, external radiation therapy to the entire abdomen to field sizes that include the lower lung fields is as effective as cytotoxic chemotherapy in achieving progression-free intervals and apparent cures. These data were developed at the M. D. Anderson Hospital in an era when cytotoxic therapy was primarily with alkylating agents, and at the Princess Margaret Hospital in Toronto during the early years of the platinum era. Many attempts at prospectively randomizing patients between cytotoxic therapy and whole abdominal radiation have been unsuccessful, both in the United States and in Canada.

The prevalent postoperative treatment has been with cytotoxic chemotherapy, and while there is controversy as to the most effective regimen and the preferred schedule or dose intensity, it can be reasonably stated that the best single cytotoxic agent for treatment of epithelial ovarian carcinoma is cisplatin or carboplatin. Other agents employed with platinum drugs include doxorubicin (Adriamycin), cyclophosphamide, hexamethylmelamine, etoposide, and, most recently, taxol. While some have argued that cisplatin or carboplatin alone are as effective as those drugs in any combination, there is accumulating data from metaanalyses suggesting that platinum combinations are superior to platinum single agents. While there has been objection to doxorubicin as being noncontributory to the various combinations, recent metaanalysis suggest a positive role for doxorubicin in the treatment of epithelial ovarian cancer. Most recently the initial experience of the Gynecological Oncology Group suggests that the combination of cisplatin and taxol is superior to that of cisplatin and cytoxan in the treatment of epithelial ovarian cancer in achieving clinical response, negative second-look laparotomies, and median duration of progression-free interval.

After initial cytoreductive surgery and aggressive treatment with a platinum-containing cytotoxic chemotherapy regimen, one should expect that at least 50% of patients with stage III and IV ovarian cancer so treated will have no identifiable disease by noninvasive testing. If one submits this group to surgical "end staging" (second look), at least half will have no histologically identifiable residual disease. The surgical second look to define tumor status after chemotherapy should be preceded by a careful laparoscopic search. Since 50% of "negative" laparoscopies miss small deposits (either microscopic or extraperitoneal), we perform immediate laparotomy under the same anesthesia. All areas where disease was known to have existed at the time of initial laparotomy are biopsied, nodes are removed, cytologic washings are taken, and a careful standard set of biopsies is taken from 30 to 50 sites.

Of the patients with residual disease, most have microscopic or very small residual disease, and approximately half of these patients can be successfully retreated with cytotoxic therapy and rendered histologically disease-free. It is thus reasonable to expect that 35% of patients with stages III and IV ovarian cancer who submit to aggressive surgery and cytotoxic therapy can be rendered histologically free of disease.

Unfortunately this does not translate to "cure," because in the experience of most treatment centers, up to 40% of these patients develop disease that is histologically identical to their original disease at some time during the 10 years following completion of therapy. Whether this rediscovered disease represents posttherapeutic residuum the virulence of which has been sufficiently altered to remain dormant or whether it represents the continued signal from oncogenes that have been unaltered and continue to signal a very large mesothelial surface (the remaining peritoneum) is impossible to discern currently. Fortunately late recurrences can often be retreated with excellent palliation and sometimes with significant extension of life.

Because receptors for estrogen and progesterone can be identified in ovarian carcinomas, there have been attempts to control this disease by the administration of progestational agents and tamoxifen. Several centers have reported a 20% clinical response rate when tamoxifen is administered to patients who have been treated without complete success for stages III and IV ovarian carcinoma. The response rate to progestational agents is less impressive. Early experiences in treating patients with passive immunostimulation by inoculation with either BCG or C. parvum suggested efficacy. However, when these agents were employed along with cytotoxic therapy in prospective studies, evidence of their utility disappeared.

More recently there is an accumulating experience with the use of cell-stimulating factors in the treatment of patients with widespread ovarian carcinoma. The main role of these biologic response modifiers would seem to lie in protecting the patients against the adverse effect of cytotoxic therapy. Except for some evidence of cytotoxic properties of interferons when given intraperitoneally, there is little evidence of other clinically effective cytotoxicity.

While the technology exists for raising antibodies to ovarian cancer antigens in animal models and complexing these antibodies with cytotoxic substances or with radionuclides and injecting them into patients with ovarian cancer, several problems diminish therapeutic utility. The presence of blocking antibodies in the patient, nonspecificity, volume of disease, geographic privilege of certain tumor deposits, and acquired human antibodies to the animal antibody all currently limit the applicability of this form of active immunotherapy.

Three issues currently engender controversy in the clinical management of patients with epithelial ovarian carcinoma; they are

1. The role of initial cytoreduction
2. The role of second-look laparotomy
3. The role of interval or secondary cytoreduction

The impact of initial cytoreduction could be studied in a randomized fashion by performing staging laparotomies and based on immediate-frozen section reports, after careful measurement of tumor bulk, randomizing patients in the operating room to cytoreductive surgery followed by cytotoxic chemotherapy or cytotoxic chemotherapy alone. Because of the experience of most gynecologic oncologists, it would be difficult in most collaborative settings to overcome the bias that favors cytoreduction and to carry out this clinical trial.

The second issue could be resolved more easily by simply randomizing one-half the patients who are eligible for a second look into an "observation only" arm; over a period of years one could determine whether treating such patients when their recurrences are discovered clinically would disadvantage them compared with those patients in whom microscopic or minimal residual disease is identified immediately and thus treated sooner. The experience in our institution based on treatment of 150 of our patients who underwent a second look compared with a group eligible for a second look who refused the procedure suggests that early identification of minimal or microscopic disease allows us to retreat those patients more successfully then waiting for their disease to manifest itself clinically. Much larger trials are necessary to resolve this issue with authority.

The final issue has been resolved in our institution and at the Memorial Sloan-Kettering Cancer Center in favor of secondary cytoreductive surgery. While the opportunity for cure is small when bulky recurrences are identified, there is a significant difference in progression-free interval and survival among those patients in whom secondary cytoreduction is performed, and thus we favor this approach.

Once a patient is thought to have been cured of ovarian cancer, close surveillance by physical examination, measurement of serum markers, and careful noninvasive radiography is required, probably for the rest of the patient's life. Early detection of rising levels of serum markers have, in our experience, been active reflections of recurrence, and retreatment employing the marker as a measurement of efficacy is useful. Future directions in this complex of diseases have already been identified. Molecular biologists are studying the gene locations associated with ovarian carcinoma, transgenic animal models have already been created for studying a variety of neoplastic processes, and hopefully, through a better understanding of the genetic signal for oncogenic transformation, interception and remedy of these defects may be possible before clinical translation destroys the host.

# 3

# Management of Nonepithelial Germ Cell and Sex Cord–Stromal Tumors of the Ovary

*Albert Altchek, M.D.*

## MANAGEMENT OF GERM CELL TUMORS OF THE OVARY

About 70% of all ovarian tumors, but about 90% of ovarian malignances, are epithelial-serous, mucinous, endometrioid, and clear cell. Therefore, the statistics of ovarian cancer are the statistics of epithelial ovarian cancer. The most common epithelial malignancy is serous, which represents 40% of ovarian malignancies. It occurs with increasing frequency with age, is usually found over the age of 40, and is usually bilateral when discovered. Because of the absence of early symptoms, it is usually discovered late with a dismal approximately 30% cure rate. This has not changed much in the past 30 years despite new chemotherapy.

Germ cell tumors are different from the common ovarian epithelial tumors. Although germ cell tumors are estimated to represent from 15 to 30% of all ovarian neoplasms, they do not represent the same proportion of malignant tumors. Germ cell tumors account for only about 1 to 5% of malignant ovarian neoplasms. The reason is that most germ cell neoplasms are benign

mature cystic teratomas, whose popular name is *dermoid cyst*.

In reviewing the management of ovarian germ cell tumors, one gets a distorted viewpoint in looking at the pathology outline listing of such tumors. Buried away in the outline is the mature cystic teratoma. It is very easy not to realize that it may represent about 95% of all germ cell tumors! This explains why only a small percentage of germ cell tumors are malignant.

Germ cell malignancies are rare, occur in the young patient, are usually unilateral, and recently have had an almost miraculous reversal of a dismal prognosis with new chemotherapy. Because of the age of the patients and the unilaterality of the tumors, efforts are made to preserve fertility.

The benign mature cystic teratoma is one of the most common ovarian neoplasms. It represents about 30% of all benign ovarian neoplasms, 30% of benign ovarian tumors, and 65% of all neoplasms under age 15.

The immature teratoma is relatively rare and malignant. Despite the similar name and cell type origin, the immature teratoma and the benign mature cyotic teratoma are very different, and this helps to understand why the gynecologist clings to the term *dermoid cyst* rather than *mature teratoma*. There is also a very rare benign solid mature teratoma that must be differentiated from the malignant solid immature teratoma.

Another disadvantage of the present outline system is that if one is not conversant with terminology, one may wonder, for example, whether the endodermal sinus tumor (also called yolk sac tumor) is benign or malignant (or for that matter, the sex cord–stromal tumor with annular tubules). Obviously, the clinician would like to have an immediate simple description—is it benign or malignant?

Therefore, perhaps pathology outlines of ovarian tumors should, in addition to traditional grouping by cell type and origin, give an estimate of incidence and whether the tumor is benign or malignant (or the chance of each). This would help with immediate clinical decisions.

The first concern with dermoids is the diagnosis. They are usually asymptomatic when small and are sometimes discovered by coincidental ultrasonography or Xray studies. They have a characteristic unilocular picture that overrides their suspicious-for-malignancy scoring on standard morphology indices because of high echogenicity and solid areas. Transvaginal color Doppler ultrasound may confirm a benign neoplasm. Their sebaceous content is liquid fat (echogenic) at body temperature, and there is often a fat-water level. They often contain a solid echogenic mural nodule (*mammillary body*) and sometimes contain teeth. They may cause acute pain with a biologic accident such as torsion and ischemic necrosis. They may be bilateral in about 10 to 15% of cases. On physical examination, the examiner may have a doughy sensation and the dermoids may float anterior to the uterus because of their liquid fat content. Dermoids tend to occur in the adolescent and young adult, and in pregnancy, although they may be present in all age groups.

Although there is no urgency in the asymptomatic patient, dermoids should be removed surgically. They are true neoplasms, usually keep growing, and may have a biologic accident. In addition, there is an overall 1 to 2% chance of secondary malignant change, usually a stratified squamous mucosa carcinoma in 75% of the transformations and adenocarcinoma in about 7%.[1] Malignant change tends to occur more often in the older patient. When the secondary squamous carcinoma has spread beyond the ovary, the prognosis is poor. "Radical surgery" is therefore considered for any dermoid cyst with local adhesion in which the possibility of malignant change is suspected.[2]

The standard method of treating dermoid cysts is by laparotomy. If possible an ovarian cystectomy is done rather than oophorectomy, thereby preserving the remaining normal ovary, which is important for the young patient. Gynecologists tend to do cystectomies while general surgeons tend to do oophorectomies, probably because of training patterns. Care is taken to avoid spillage of the contents, which are irritating and can cause a chemical peritonitis with severe adhesions if not removed. The resected dermoid cyst is sent to the pathology department for a frozen section to verify the diagnosis and be certain that there is no secondary malignant change.

If there is a secondary malignant change, then an ipsilateral salpingo-oophorectomy is done, as well as a biopsy of the opposite ovary and a surgical staging laparotomy. For the patient in whom childbearing is of no concern, a total abdominal hysterectomy and bilateral salpingo-oophorectomy (BSO) are done. For the young patient desiring to retain fertility, an unaffected opposite ovary and the uterus may be left in situ.

Even if the dermoid cyst has no secondary malignant change in the postmenopausal woman, a total abdominal hysterectomy and BSO are often done. If there is no malignant change in the dermoid cyst, and if the residual fragile fragment of ipsilateral normal ovary is to be preserved it is carefully examined for hemostasis, which may be difficult since it may contain large blood vessels. Most gynecologists use fine absorbable synthetic sutures for hemostasis and to close the dead space and then approximate the edges of the residual ovary with running or running locked sutures. Keeping the surface suture material to a minimum may reduce adhesion formation. Oxidized cellulose (Interceed) may be used to cover the ovary for the same purpose. Surgeons have left Hyskon in the peritoneal cavity to reduce adhesions, but this may cause allergic or anaphylactic reactions. Lactated Ringer's solution with or without heparin has also been left intraperitoneally. A microsurgical philosophy of minimum injury is desirable.

In the past with benign dermoids, the opposite ovary was bisected to look for a small dermoid. This is avoided at present if the opposite ovary is normal on inspection and palpation to avoid adhesion formation and because the yield is small.

The traditional standard abdominal incision is a lower abdominal midline vertical or paramedian incision. The advantage is that the preoperative diagnosis may be uncertain. In addition, if unexpectedly there is a secondary malignant change, then surgical staging is feasible.

Some surgeons use a lower abdominal transverse incision (Pfannenstiel) if they believe the diagnosis is a dermoid cyst and if the patient is very anxious to avoid a vertical scar. Should there be an unexpected malignancy, the incision may have to be extended upward.

In recent years with advanced laparoscopy technology, some gynecologists have been removing dermoid cysts (cystectomy) by laparoscopy. Small cysts are removed intact with a bag through the laparoscopy port or by pulling it through an abdominal stab incision. Larger dermoid cysts are removed in pieces or through a posterior colposcopy incision. The potential problems with laparoscopy are spillage of irritating contents, misdiagnosis of a malignant cyst, and lack of recognition of a secondary malignant change. There are differences of opinion regarding the use of laparoscopy itself and the size of dermoid cysts to be removed. Although spillage of irritating contents is known to cause a severe chemical peritonitis and adhesions, it may be that this applies to spontaneous rupture with intraperitoneal retention of the contents. Apparently with surgical leakage and immediate irrigation and cleansing, there is less chance of peritoneal irritation.

## MALIGNANT OVARIAN GERM CELL NEOPLASMS

Williams and Gershenson[3] and others[4–7] have recently reviewed the management of malignant ovarian germ cell neoplasms. Because these tumors are different from each other, because they are rare and therefore experience is limited, and because of the recent development of chemotherapy to which they are exquisitely sensitive, a somewhat detailed review of new concepts will be presented.

Malignant germ cell tumors are very different from malignant epithelial cell tumors in incidence, epidemiology, biology, and management. Germ cell tumors constitute only about 5% of malignant ovarian tumors compared with about 90% epithelial depending on the age group. In younger patients the percent of germ cell malignant tumors is increased while that of epithelial cancers is decreased. Although oral contraceptive use and pregnancy significantly reduce the risk of epithelial ovarian cancer, these factors have no clear effect on germ cell or stromal ovarian cancers.[8] While overexpression of the *ras* oncogene product p21 is increased in malignant compared with benign ovarian epithelial neoplasms, increased overexpression is not found in germ cell and sex cord–stromal neoplasms. This suggests a different histiogenesis and different carcinogenic mechanism.[9] Germ cell tumors tend to occur in adolescents and young adults. They are rapidly growing and used to have a very poor prognosis, although with dysgerminoma, radiation therapy gave good results for recurrences. Recently, there has been an extraordinary change. Radiation is rarely used since it is not desirable in young persons and since it may destroy ovarian func-

tion. New and very effective chemotherapy has been developed with a reversal from poor to good prognosis. With epithelial tumors, despite new platinum chemotherapy and despite good immediate results, the increase in survival has been only marginal.

Germ cell tumors are usually unilateral even with metastatic spread. Prophylactic removal of the opposite uninvolved ovary and uninvolved uterus does not improve results. Since these tumors often occur in young persons, it is often possible to do a unilateral salpingo-oophorectomy. Even with advanced disease with debulking and node surgery and chemotherapy, future childbearing may be possible.[10] With germ cell tumors, even if the opposite ovary is involved, the uterus may still be able to be preserved, which still permits future fertility with ovum donation and an in vitro fertilization. Germ cell tumors have more reliable serum markers than epithelial tumors. Germ cell tumors are less aggressively debulked, reliance being made on chemotherapy. It is relatively unusual to perform second-look surgery for germ cell tumors.

At the University of Texas M. D. Anderson Cancer Center, the age for malignant ovarian germ cell tumors ranged from 6 to 46 years with a median age of 16 to 20 years.[3] The occurrence with pregnancy is simply an overlap with young age. About 85% present with abdominal pain and a palpable mass, and about 10% have acute pain due to a biologic accident. In the child and young adolescent, ovarian tumors are abdominal rather than pelvic, and acute symptoms tend to progress rapidly. Less common subacute signs include abdominal distension, vaginal bleeding, fever, and pseudoprecocious puberty.

Serum markers may be helpful with diagnosis and monitoring. Characteristically, endodermal sinus tumor produces α-fetoprotein (AFP) and choriocarcinoma produces human chorionic gonadotropin (HCG). Kawai et al. reported that (AFP) levels were elevated in all yolk sac (endodermal sinus) tumors, in about 60% of immature teratomas, and in about 12% of dysgerminomas.[11] AFP levels were over 1000 mg/ml in 34 of 36 yolk sac tumors, but less than that in 20 of 21 immature teratomas. The AFP cutoff value was 20 ng/ml. The Ca 125 cutoff value was 35 μ/ml. The Ca 125 test was positive in 12 of 12 yolk sac tumors, and in 10 of 12 immature teratomas. Dysgerminomas and mature cystic teratomas with malignant transformation had a 55% positive rate. Mature cystic teratomas had a positive rate of 23.7%. Ca 125 was considered a screening marker for malignancy in germ cell tumors, and Ca 125 levels can be elevated in any of them. The Ca 19-9 cutoff was 37 μ/ml. About half of all malignant and benign teratomas show elevations of Ca 19-9 levels. The lactate dehydrogenase (LDH) cutoff was 450 Iu/l. The LDH level was elevated in 19 of 20 cases of dysgerminoma, often with a very high level of over 1000 Iu/l (mean 1910 Iu/l). The LDH level was increased in 10 of 12 cases of yolk sac tumor (mean 634 Iu/l). The level of the normal or H isoenzyme of LDH is elevated in dysgerminoma, while epithelial cancer is inclined to elevations in levels of sub-unit M.

Tissue polypeptide antigen (TPA, cutoff value 110 μ/l) and carcinoembryonic antigen (CEA, cutoff value 5 ng/ml) were not considered useful tumor markers for germ cell tumors.

If HCG is present, it indicates syncytiotrophoblastic giant cells in a yolk sac tumor or dysgerminoma.

Therefore, elevation of AFP levels is helpful in suggesting and differentiating between yolk sac tumors and immature teratomas. In general, elevated Ca 125 levels suggest a malignant germ cell tumor. An elevated LDH level suggests a dysgerminoma, while an elevated Ca 19-9 level suggests a teratomatous tumor.[11]

Aside from the previously unrecognized LDH level elevation, dysgerminomas may have increases in neuron-specific enolase and HCG levels.[3]

Since malignant germ cell tumors are very rare, serum tumor marker screening is not done. Serum tests may be helpful after clinical discovery in suggesting a preoperative diagnosis. Serum tests may also be helpful in monitoring therapy. The first report of serial LDH measurements to detect recurrence in ovarian dysgerminoma was made in 1992,[12] although previously AFP elevation had been found with endodermal sinus tumors and HCG elevation had been found with choriocarcinomas.

After clinical discovery of a malignant germ cell tumor, the ultrasound image is that of a large solid neoplasm, sometimes with areas of cystic liquefaction breakdown. Color Doppler waveform analysis should suggest a malignant pattern. Although there should be appropriate clinical indications for surgery, preparation should be made for a cancer approach, (such as vertical incision, peritoneal washings, frozen section, oncology consultation, possible node dissection, tumor debulking, omentectomy, etc).

The main function of ultrasonography would be to show a characteristic benign cystic mature teratoma (dermoid cyst).

Malignant ovarian germ cell tumors are large at discovery, with a median size of 16 cm and a range of 7 to 40 cm.[3] This suggests a lack of early symptoms, and rapid growth. With dysgerminomas, there may be a 10% chance of gross bilaterality and a 10% chance of microscopic bilaterality. With other malignant germ cell tumors, bilaterality is very rare, in the range of 1% or less. If there is bilaterality, it may indicate a mixed tumor with dysgerminoma or an advanced stage of any

malignant germ cell tumor. With endodermal sinus tumor and immature teratoma, a benign cystic mature teratoma (dermoid cyst) may occur in about 10% of cases, which may confuse the clinical presentation. "Benign cystic teratoma is associated with 5 to 10% of malignant germ cell tumors" and can be found in the ipsilateral, contralateral, or bilateral ovary locations.[3] Preexisting gonadoblastoma may also be present, especially with an abnormal gonad and a Y chromosome.

Personal speculation is that the presence of a dermoid and gonadoblastoma suggests an inherent susceptibility to germ cell tumor formation. This might be compared with first-degree relatives of epithelial ovarian cancer patients; these relatives have an increased incidence of ovarian cancer but also have an increase in benign and bilateral neoplasms.[13]

Ascites and tumor rupture (because of its friable nature), each occur in about 20% of cases of malignant germ cell tumors.

Whereas the frequent epithelial cancer frequently spreads via the peritoneum and, apparently less often, the lymph nodes, the malignant germ cell tumor apparently spreads more through the nodes (and hematogenously to the liver and lung) than does the epithelial. Whereas epithelial cancer is usually found in stage III, germ cell cancer usually is in stage I in 60 to 70% and stage III in 25 to 30%. Stage II (pelvic extension) and stage IV (distant metastases) are unusual at discovery.

With a large solid ovarian mass and symptoms, surgery becomes a relatively urgent matter. The surgeon should be knowledgable with pertinent clinical aspects.

A vertical lower abdominal incision is made. If the tumor seems benign (dermoid), then an ovarian cystectomy is done with an immediate frozen section. If the tumor appears malignant grossly (or is found to be malignant after cystectomy), then a unilateral salpingo-oophorectomy (USO) is done. If the neoplasm is dysgerminoma, the opposite ovary is biopsied and if positive or if it is a dysgenetic gonad, then a BSO is done with preservation of the uninvolved uterus. This is different from an older recommendation for hysterectomy in addition to BSO. At present, with assisted reproductive technology, pregnancy is possible with a uterus, without ovaries, using ovum donation and in vitro fertilization. One investigator as a research study has not removed the opposite ovary with microscopic dysgerminoma, relying on chemotherapy.

If the opposite ovary contains a benign dermoid cyst, then a cystectomy is done with preservation of residual normal ovarian tissue.

If the tumor is a nondysgerminomatous malignant germ cell tumor and the opposite ovary appears grossly normal, it is not biopsied, because the chance of bilaterality is about only 1%, because it does not improve the prognosis if the biopsy is negative, and to avoid adhesions that may interfere with future fertility.

If the neoplasm is apparently confined to one or both ovaries, then surgical staging is done to be certain that the tumor is not in a more advanced stage that will affect the prognosis and later possible chemotherapy.

The surgical staging is similar to that of the common epithelial ovarian cancers. Ascitic fluid or peritoneal washings are studied. The entire peritoneal surface is visualized and palpated. Any obvious tumor masses or enlarged nodes are removed or biopsied. If no obvious neoplasm spread is found, then multiple peritoneal biopsies are done of sites prone to metastases and of the omentum as well as sampling of pelvic and paraaortic lymph nodes. There is no therapeutic value to complete node dissection or very aggressive debulking of tumor. Bowel is not usually resected for serosal implants. The essential treatment is prompt chemotherapy, since malignant germ cell tumors are much more sensitive to such therapy than the common epithelial tumors, as well rapid-growing.

If the patient was not adequately surgically staged with the initial surgery and if the neoplasm is a usually chemosensitive tumor, then repeat surgery for staging is usually not done since chemotherapy will be used. Noninvasive evaluation such as ultrasonography, computerized axial tomography, and serum markers is used.[3]

Prior to chemotherapy most nondysgerminomatous malignant germ cell tumors were rapidly fatal. With prompt chemotherapy, the prognosis has been reversed. With early-stage completely resected nondysgerminomatous tumors and cisplatin-based chemotherapy, probably all can be cured. Even with advanced cancer about 65% can be cured.

Regarding chemotherapy, "most investigators feel that the combination of cisplatin, etoposide, and bleomycin (BEP) is the preferred regimen."[3A] Chemotherapy use requires experience, since there may be a 1% mortality with febrile neutropenic episodes. Cisplatin may cause nephrotoxicity, and bleomycin can cause pulmonary fibrosis. The previous standard chemotherapy had been vincristine, dactinomycin, and cyclophosphamide (VAC); however, BEP is superior in efficacy, and etoposide is less toxic than vinblastine.

Among nondysgerminomatous tumors, there is a 75% recurrence rate with resected stage I endodermal sinus tumor, embryonal carcinoma, mixed germ cell tumor, and grade 3 immature teratoma! This attests to the inherent aggressiveness of these malignancies. "Thus, all patients except those with grade I, stage I immature teratoma should receive adjuvant chemotherapy."[3B]

Although current chemotherapy was originally developed for use with malignant testicular germ cell tumors, there are differences in usage. With testicular tumors, adjuvant chemotherapy may be deferred, while ovarian tumors recur more rapidly and have a poorer prognosis. Therefore, chemotherapy is begun within a week of surgery regardless of serum markers.

If tumors are initially sensitive to chemotherapy but then recur, then combination therapy with cisplatin, vinblastine, and ifosfamide is considered.

If tumors are resistant, then high-dose chemotherapy and bone marrow rescue are considered.

The second-look laparotomy was developed to examine chemotherapy-treated epithelial cancer cases without clinical evidence of disease. For malignant germ cell tumors, second-look laparotomy may not be necessary since it is usually negative. It is not done for dysgerminoma.

With early-stage nondysgerminoma germ cell tumors, second-look laparotomy is not done. For those with originally advanced disease, it may occasionally be done.

If there is a residual mass after chemotherapy, it is usually fibrosis or rarely a mature teratoma following a previous immature teratoma. The options include second-look laparotomy, fine-needle biopsy, or surveillance with imaging and serum markers. Current opinion favors trying to avoid laparotomy.

In a personal unpublished case of an infant with an endodermal sinus tumor of the upper vagina and extensive retroperitoneal node involvement, there was a loss of ultrasound color flow in the residual mass, which at laparotomy was found not to contain viable tumor. Disappearance of ultrasound color flow may in the future be another method aside from AFP of determining whether a residual mass is fibrosis or tumor.

Dysgerminomas are the most common malignant germ cell tumors and account for 50% of all malignant germ cell tumors. They are tumors of adolescence, young adulthood, and pregnancy, with an age range of 4 to 50 years. They are lobulated, firm, fleshy, pale tan tumors. They are different from other ovarian malignant germ cell tumors in that they may be bilateral, are radiosensitive, and are less aggressive. The other malignant germ cell tumors include endodermal sinus tumor (yolk sac tumor), immature teratoma, embryonal carcinoma, choriocarcinoma, and mixed primitive germ cell tumors.

About 65 to 85% of dysgerminomas will be found to have the tumor in only one ovary. About 10% have gross spread, and 10% have microscopic metastases to the opposite ovary.

Until recently postoperative radiation therapy was used because dysgerminomas are very sensitive to radiation. Although effective, this treatment induced sterility. At present, chemotherapy is preferred to radiotherapy. Without radiation and with resection of ovarian disease, there may be a 15 to 25% recurrence.

For stage Ia tumors, the chance of recurrence is about 15 to 20%, and either the patient is followed or adjuvant chemotherapy is given. If the observed patient develops a recurrence, then chemotherapy is used.

The current recommendation for resected dysgerminoma stages Ib to III is three courses of BEP adjuvant chemotherapy.

Although there has not been adequate long-term follow-up, chemotherapy seems relatively safe, and in the main, ovarian function of the remaining ovary and fertility have been preserved. There may be mild peripheral neuropathy and Raynaud's phenomenon.

To retain the fertility potential, a microsurgical philosophy is used to reduce postoperative adhesion formation, the opposite uninvolved ovary and uninvolved uterus are preserved, and radiation is avoided.

With advanced-stage dysgerminoma, there is a "reasonable attempt at surgical debulking," avoiding major bowel resection, and preserving reproductive capability if feasible and appropriate. "Likewise, a procedure done specifically for debulking when the diagnosis has been established and the primary tumor removed does not seem warranted."[14] Even with advanced-stage dysgerminoma, "Chemotherapy should replace radiation as the preferred treatment in patients with resected disease selected for adjuvant treatment, particularly if fertility is an issue."[14] Three courses of BEP should be given, and the cure rate should be near 100% with acceptable morbidity.[14] "It is clear that second look laparotomy is not indicated."[14] Most favor observation of residual masses, especially if less than 3 cm. Others agree that a second look is not indicated in all cases with dysgerminoma and early-stage nondysgerminoma.[3]

Although testicular seminoma flow cytometry nuclear DNA ploidy has prognostic significance, with ovarian dysgerminoma, a homologous neoplasm, there is no prognostic significance.[15]

Despite the fact that the serum AFP level is considered a reliable marker for the management of endodermal sinus tumors, with a large, necrotic, nonviable residual tumor mass, the AFP level may remain elevated and may be misleading.[16]

With immature teratomas of the ovary, stage I, it is important to distinguish between grades 1 and 2 regarding the need for chemotherapy. Grade 1 tumors "had only a slight tendency to metastasize, whereas high grade (grade 2 and 3) tumors metastasized more frequently."[17] Therefore, there must be adequate sampling, immature neuroectoderm needs to be recognized, a reproducible semiqualitative estimate of the amount must be made, and a uniform microscopic field is required.[17]

Second-look laparotomy in germ cell tumors is not necessary in well-staged patients, surgically without evidence of disease prior to chemotherapy, and in those without teratomatous elements in the original tumor. Those with teratomatous elements and incompletely removed tumor who normalize tumor markers after chemotherapy benefit from a second look and resection of residual malignancy.[18]

On an optimistic note, "Virtually all patients with early stage, completely resected tumors other than dysgerminoma will survive after careful surgical staging and cisplatin-based adjuvant chemotherapy. In addition, over 50% to perhaps as high as 80% of patients with advanced disease will also survive their disease."[3]

## MANAGEMENT OF SEX CORD–STROMAL TUMORS OF THE OVARY

Jones,[19] Hoskins and Rubin,[20] Price and Schwartz,[21] Scully,[22] and others have written excellent reviews of sex cord–stromal tumors of the ovary. They are rare, accounting for about 6% of all ovarian neoplasms and about 7% of ovarian malignancies.[20] In addition, because of many histologic types and variations, they may be difficult to diagnose. When slides are reviewed by experienced pathologists, diagnoses are not infrequently changed. Furthermore, the frequent lack of surgical staging, lack of standard therapy, lack of follow-up, and wide age variation tend to cause confusion in prognosis and management. Of all ovarian neoplasms, the majority of endocrinologically active ones are in this group. Individual cases may be confusing since the same cell types may be estrogenic, androgenic, or inactive.

Nevertheless, there are some guidelines. In general, the sex cord–origin tumors such as the granulosa (the most common of the group) are low-grade, slow-growing malignant tumors, while the stromal-origin tumors such as the fibroma and thecoma are benign.

Sex cord–stromal tumors have also been referred to as sex cord–mesenchyme tumors, mesenchymomas, gonadal stromal tumors, and stromal tumors.[22] They include all neoplasms that derive from the sex cords (primitive cortical lobules from the coelomic epithelium) and the specialized stroma (mesenchyme) of the developing gonad. They are classified according to their histologic appearance, usually as[19]

1. Granulosa cell tumor
2. Thecoma
3. Fibroma
4. Unclassified thecoma-fibroma, sclerosing stromal
5. Sertoli–Leydig cell tumors (androblastomas)

6. Gynandroblastoma
7. Unclassified sex cord–stromal tumors
8. Sex cord tumor with annular tubules

Management of sex cord–stromal tumors of the ovary requires a frozen section done by an experienced pathologist because of innumerable varieties of rare neoplasms and difficulty in histologic diagnosis, and therefore surgery is best done during regular hours. If the tumor appears benign, it may be shelled out of its ovary for frozen section. If it seems malignant, the entire tumor and its ovary and perhaps the ipsilateral tube as well should be removed for frozen section.

If the patient is postmenopausal, a total abdominal hysterectomy and BSO are considered.

If preservation of fertility is desired, then depending on the frozen section report, the opposite ovary might be biopsied, and only a USO is considered. Over 95% of sex cord–stromal tumors are unilateral. For malignant neoplasms, ideally, through a vertical incision surgical staging is done at the same time to determine whether there is a more advanced stage regardless of whether conservative or more extensive surgery is done. Excision or debulking is done for gross neoplasm. Oncologic consultation is desirable. Endometrial sampling is done if the uterus is preserved.

Recurrences are managed surgically if possible. Residual tumor in the pelvis may be treated with radiotherapy. Chemotherapy has not been satisfactory because of the rarity of cases and only modest results in the past. It requires individualization with newer combination drugs. Radiation is considered for localized pelvic recurrent disease.

## GRANULOSA CELL TUMORS

Granulosa cell tumors account for 70% of sex cord–stromal tumors and are the most common endocrine-functioning tumor. They can occur at any age from the prepubertal child to the 70-year-old woman, with a peak in the perimenopause, at about age 52.[20] Although they constitute less than 2% of all ovarian neoplasms, they account for 6% of ovarian cancers. About 95% are adult (rather than juvenile) granulosa cell tumors.[20]

Granulosa cell tumors have also been called granulosa–theca cell tumor, feminizing mesenchymoma, gynoblastoma, and follicular and granulosa cell carcinoma.[22]

The gross appearance of the granulosa cell tumor varies from a soft or firm solid gray, yellow, or white tumor to a multicystic (with a watery fluid or blood) semisolid tumor, or infrequently to a uni- or multilocular cystic mass with thin-walled compartments containing watery fluid. The granulosa cell tumor is suscep-

tible to spontaneous or intraoperative rupture.[22] Most are solid with cystic areas of hemorrhage and necrosis.[19]

Over 95% of granulosa cell tumors are unilateral with an average size of 12 cm. About 90% are stage I.[19]

When granulosa cell tumors occur in children and young adults, there is a 90% chance they will have a distinct histologic appearance with large, immature disorderly cells, and these tumors are referred to as juvenile granulosa cell tumors.

When granulosa cell tumors occur in the prepubertal girl, about 75% of the girls experience pseudoprecocious puberty due to estrogen secretion.[22A]

In the menstruating woman, granulosa cell tumors may cause amenorrhea, often followed by and sometimes only with irregular bleeding. The endometrium may show cystic glandular hyperplasia due to unopposed estrogen stimulation. Sometimes, there is adenomatous hyperplasia, which may become atypical and progress to endometrial adenocarcinoma.[22B]

In the postmenopausal woman, granulosa cell tumors cause uterine bleeding, endometrial atypical hyperplasia, and endometrial adenocarcinoma in 5 to 25% of patients. These cancers are usually low-grade and rarely metastasize.[22B]

Granulosa cell tumors cause an estrogenic vaginal smear with a preponderance of superficial cells.

Aside from their estrogenic effects, there may be nonspecific presentations of ascites in 10%; rarely pleural effusion (Meigs's syndrome); hematoperitoneum in 5 to 20% due to rupture; tumor mass; acute pain; local contiguous spread; and uterine fibroids.

Clinically, the granulosa cell tumor is of low-grade malignancy. Recurrences may occur 5 to 20 years after surgery and tend to remain in the pelvis or abdomen. Hematologic metastases are very rare, may occur after many years, and may appear in the lungs, liver, bone, and brain.[22C] Some believe that granulosa cell tumors spread like common epithelial cancers via the peritoneum, local extension, and lymphatic and hematogenous routes; however, there is a preference for the last two. Most agree that they have slow growth and late recurrences.

There have been a few granulosa cell tumors that virilize, and these tend to have the rare gross pathologic appearance of a large unilocular or multilocular thin-walled cyst.[22C]

The usual management is total abdominal hysterectomy and BSO. If it is desired to preserve fertility and if the tumor is only in one ovary and contained in the capsule, then the opposite ovary is biopsied and surgical staging is done. Under such circumstances a USO and endometrial sampling are done and the patient is followed for the rest of her life.

For stage IC tumors with the tumor confined to one ovary and with rupture pre- or intraoperatively, if surgical staging does not reveal further extension and if fertility is desired, then in addition to USO and endometrial sampling, three cycles of BEP chemotherapy are given.

Postoperative adjuvant chemotherapy is controversial. At Yale, BEP is offered to women with stage Ia granulosa cell tumors over age 40, and to all women with stages Ib to IV. Patients are followed at 3-month intervals for the first year, at 4-month intervals for the second year, at 6-month intervals to the fifth year, and then annually. An annual chest x-ray examination is done. Computed tomography (CT) scan is done after therapy as a baseline. Second-look laparotomy is not routine.[21A]

For tumor rupture, advanced-stage, unresectable, and recurrent tumors, chemotherapy with cisplatin, vinblastine, and bleomycin (BVC) has been used with a response rate of about 50% but with dangerous toxicity. As with germ cell tumors, etoposide is now being used instead of vinblastine (BEP) to reduce toxicity. Studies of the latter are in progress.[21]

It must be remembered that cancer chemotherapy requires experience, that recommendations may change with time, and that "the optimal chemotherapeutic regimen for treating advanced and recurrent granulosa cell tumors remains to be established."[19A]

Serum tumor markers may be of value (if their levels have been found to be elevated) in monitoring and include estradiol, follicle regulatory protein, and inhibin.[23]

Recurrences may occur within 2 years or many years later so that the survival rate for 5 years is about 85%, 10 years 70%, and 20 years 50%. Therefore, all cases are observed indefinitely.

Although the behavior of the individual tumor is usually unpredictable, suggestions of poor prognosis include advanced stage, size over 5 cm, tumor rupture, high grade, age over 40 years, and especially recurrent disease.

It is uncertain whether a large size of tumor, of itself, is important or whether a large tumor may be associated with unrecognized spread.

### Juvenile Granulosa Cell Tumors

About 5% of all granulosa cell tumors are juvenile granulosa cell tumors, so-named both because they occur in the young patient, usually under age 20, and because of less differentiation. They account for 5 to 12% of ovarian tumors in the child and adolescent. They have an ominous histologic appearance with marked nuclear atypia and high mitotic activity. Understandably, they cause isosexual pseudoprecocious puberty. They may rarely be associated with Ollier's disease (enchondro-

matosis), Maffucci's syndrome (enchondromatosis and hemangiomas), abnormal chromosomes, and ambiguous external genitalia.

Juvenile granulosa cell tumors are usually unilateral, large, solid with cystic portions, and stage I.

Since the patient is usually young and since the tumor is usually stage I, the usual treatment is USO with surgical staging and endometrial sampling. Advanced-stage disease requires more surgery. Cisplatin, doxorubicin, and cyclophosphamide (CAP), PVP, BEP, and methotrexate, actinomycin D, and chlorambucil (MAC)[24] have been used for combination chemotherapy, but BEP is being used mainly at present.

Despite the ominous histologic appearance, the cure rate for stage I disease is 93 to 95% by surgery. Advanced-stage disease has a poor prognosis. The stage at discovery is the most reliable prognostic sign. Unlike the adult slow-growing recurrences, juvenile recurrences are often within 3 years.

Since the histologic appearance is not a reliable guide to prognosis, DNA ploidy has been investigated. No association was found between DNA ploidy and survival with stage Ia juvenile granulosa cell tumors of the ovary.[25] There was a suggestion that DNA ploidy and mean S-phase fraction might show an association with stage III tumors.

## THECOMA AND FIBROMA TUMORS

### THECOMA TUMORS

Thecoma tumors are generally benign and occur in older patients. Thecomas cause only 1% of all ovarian neoplasms; are usually unilateral, large, solid, and benign; occur at an average age of 53; and may secrete estrogen.

The usual treatment for postmenopausal women is hysterectomy and BSO. To preserve fertility, oophorectomy or salpingo-oophorectomy is done. The tumor does not have a capsule but is well delineated. There may be endometrial hyperplasia or neoplasia, and therefore uterine curettage is done.

### FIBROMA TUMORS

Ovarian fibromas cause 4% of all ovarian neoplasms and are considered by some to be the most common sex cord–stromal tumor.[19] They tend to occur in adults and are solid, unilateral, and benign. About 1% of fibromas are accompanied by Meigs's syndrome of ascites and pleural effusion. Rarely, there may be Gorlin's syndrome of bilateral tumors with basal cell nevi.

Very rarely, there may be cellular fibromas with one to three mitotic figures per 10 high-power fields and only slight nuclear atypia, which are considered of LMP. Those with four or more mitotic figures with nuclear atypia are considered to be malignant fibrosarcoma.

## STROMAL TUMOR WITH MINOR SEX CORD ELEMENTS

The stromal tumor with minor sex cord elements is a rare benign thecoma-fibroma containing sex cord derivations. Some develop collagenous sclerosis (sclerosing stromal tumor).

## SERTOLI–STROMAL CELL TUMORS

Sertoli cell tumors may be estrogenic in 70% of cases and androgenic in 20%. There is confusion in terminology because *androblastoma* is used for both Sertoli and Leydig cell tumors.

Sertoli cell tumors are benign, unilateral, solid, and usually less than 5 cm.

## LEYDIG CELL TUMORS

Leydig cell tumors are rare, 80% benign androgenic and 10% estrogenic. Most occur between ages 50 and 60, but they can occur at any age. They are small at discovery because their endocrine activity invites investigation. They can secrete testosterone even when small and difficult to discover.

Histologically, most are hilus tumor cells, with Leydig tumor cells less frequent, but their clinical presentation and management are similar. They are usually benign, unilateral, less than 5 cm, not encapsulated but well outlined, and soft-solid.

To preserve fertility, oophorectomy is done. After menopause, hysterectomy and BSO are advised. There may be endometrial stimulation.

## SERTOLI–LEYDIG CELL TUMORS

Sertoli–Leydig cell tumors are also called androblastomas and arrhenoblastomas because about half cause androgenic effects with elevated levels of serum testosterone. They number less than 0.5% of all ovarian neoplasms. Another tumor marker may be AFP.

The well-differentiated form is also called *tubular adenoma of Pick* and is unilateral, of 5 cm average size, firm, and lobulated.

Most Sertoli–Leydig cell tumors are intermediately differentiated, found at an average age of 25 years, and solid-cystic with an average size of 10 cm.

There may be poorly differentiated tumors and those with heterologus elements.

For the older or postmenopausal patient, abdominal hysterectomy and BSO are advised.

For the younger woman who wishes to remain fertile, a USO is done if the neoplasm is well or intermediately differentiated and is confined to one ovary (stage Ia1).

If the tumor is poorly differentiated, then hysterectomy with BSO and adjuvant chemotherapy are planned.

The prognosis depends on stage and grade with well-differentiated stage Ia1 acting like benign tumors.

Intermediately differentiated neoplasms have a 3 to 11% chance of malignancy with adverse factors being rupture and histologic retiform pattern and heterologous mesenchymal elements.

Poorly differentiated neoplasms have an over 50% chance of being malignant.

Recurrences may appear within 3 years and have a poor prognosis. Conventional radiotherapy and chemotherapy are not effective. BEP chemotherapy is being investigated.[19]

## GYNANDROBLASTOMA

Gynoblastomas may cause androgen or estrogen excess or be hormonally inactive. They are usually unilateral, solid, small, and benign. Histologically, there are granulosa and Sertoli-Leydig cells.

## SEX CORD TUMOR WITH ANNULAR TUBULES

Sex cord tumors with annuler tubules (SCTATs) often occur in association with Peutz-Jeghers syndrome (P-JS) of perioral melanin pigmentation and intestinal polyposis (see the section on genetic aspects in Chapter 1).

Most women with P-JS have ovarian SCTAT. The mean age is 27, and half the tumors are estrogenic. SCTATs are bilateral in two-thirds of the patients and appear as small nodules 3 cm or less. Although the SCTAT itself is benign, it may be a marker for a malignant adenocarcinoma of the endocervix (adenoma malignum) and possibly breast cancer.

With SCTAT without P-JS, the SCTAT is usually unilateral, solid with cystic degeneration, and larger, and about half the tumors are estrogenic.

About 20% of SCTAT are clinically malignant, as opposed to SCTAT with P-JS with a benign course. For the older patient, hysterectomy and BSO are advised. For the young patient, a USO is done if the tumor is confined to the one ovary. Tumor masses are resected therapeutically without reliance on chemotherapy.

# REFERENCES

1. Ueda G, Fujita M, Ogawa H, Sawada M, Inoue M, Tanizawa O. Adenocarcinoma in a benign cystic teratoma of the ovary: Report of a case with a long survival period. *Gynecol Oncol* 48:259–263, 1993.

2. Hudson CN, Shepard JH. Surgery for carcinoma of ovary. In *Gynecologic Oncology, Fundamental Principles and Clinical Practice,* 2d ed, Coppleson M, Monaghan JM, Morrow CP, Tattersall MHN, eds. New York, Churchill Livingstone, 1992, vol 2 pp 1313–1323.

3. Williams SD, Gershenson DM, Management of germ cell tumors of the ovary. In *Cancer of the Ovary,* Markman M, Hoskins WJ, New York, Raven Press, 1993, pp 375–384, p 378 (3A) p 379 (3B).

4. Williams SD, Gershenson DM, Horowitz CJ, Scully RE. Ovarian germ cell and stromal tumors. In *Principles and Practice of Gynecologic Oncology,* Hoskins WJ, Perez CA, Young RC, eds. Philadelphia, Lippincott, 1992, pp 715–730.

5. Gershenson DM. Malignant germ cell tumors of Ovary: Clinical Features and Management. In *Gynecologic Oncology, Fundamental Principles and Clinical Practice,* 2d ed, Coppleson M, Monaghan GM, Morrow CP, Tattersall MHN, eds. New York, Churchill Livingstone, 1992, pp 935–945.

6. Williams SD. Ovarian germ cell tumors. In *Ovarian Cancer,* Rubin SC, Sutton GP, eds. New York, McGraw-Hill, 1993, pp 391–404.

7. DiSaia P, Creasman WT. Germ cell, stromal and other ovarian tumors. In *Clinical Gynecologic Oncology,* 4th ed. St. Louis, Mosby Year Book, 1993, pp 426–457.

8. Horn-Ross PL, Whittemore AS, Harris R, Itnyre J, Collaborative Ovarian Cancer Group. Characteristics relating to ovarian cancer risk: Collaborative analysis of 12 US. case control studies: VI. Nonepithelial cancers among adults. *Epidemiology* 3:490–495, 1992.

9. Yaginuma Y, Yamashita K, Kuzumaki N, Fujita M, Shimazu T, pas Oncogene product p 21 expression and prog-

nosis or human ovarian tumors. *Gynecol Oncol* 46:45–50, 1992.

10. Wu PC, Huang RL, Lang JH, Huang HF, Lian LJ, Tang MY. Treatment of malignant ovarian germ cell tumors with preservation of fertility: A report of 28 cases. *Gynecol Oncol* 40:2–6, 1991.

11. Kawai M, Kano T, Kikkawa F, et al. Seven tumor markers in benign and malignant germ cell tumors of the ovary. *Gynecol Oncol* 45:248–253, 1992.

12. Pressley RH, Muntz HG, Falkenberry S, Rice LW. Case report: Serum lactic dehydrogenase as a tumor marker in dysgerminoma. *Gynecol Oncol* 44:281–283, 1992.

13. Boyrne TH, Whitehead ML, Campbell S, et al. Ultrasound screening for familial ovarian cancer. *Gynecol Oncol* 43:92–97, 1991.

14. Williams SD, Blessing JA, Hatch KD, Homesley HD. Chemotherapy of advanced dysgerminoma: Trials of the Gynecologic Oncology Group. *J Clin Oncol* 9:1950–1955, 1991.

15. Palmquist MB, Webb MJ, Lieber MM, Gaffey TA, Nativ O. DNA ploidy of ovarian dysgerminomas: Correlation with clinical outcome. *Gynecol Oncol* 44:13–16, 1992.

16. Whelan JS, Stebbings W, Owen RA, Chir B, Calne R, Clark PI. Successful treatment of a primary endodermal sinus tumor of the liver. *Cancer* 70:2260–2262, 1992.

17. O'Connor D, Norris H. Immature teratomas of the ovary. 24th Annual Meeting Society of Gynecologic Oncologists, February 7–10, 1993, Palm Desert, California. Abstract 1 Gyn Oncol 49:107, 1993.

18. Williams S, Blessing J, DiSaia P, Major F, Ball H. Second-look laparotomy in ovarian germ cell tumors: The Gynecologic Oncology Group (GOG) Experience. 24th Annual Meeting Society of Gynecologic Oncologists, February 7–10, 1993, Palm Desert, California. Abstract 2 Gyn Oncol 49:107, 1993.

19. Jones W. Sex Cord–Stromal Tumors of the Ovary. In *Cancer of the Ovary.* Markman M, Hoskins WJ, eds. New York, Raven, 1993. pp 385–405, p 388 (19A).

20. Hoskins WJ, Rubin SC. Malignant gonadal stromal tumors of ovary: Clinical features and management. In *Gynecologic Oncology, Fundamental Principles and Clinical Practice,* 2d ed, Coppleson M, Monaghan JM, Morrow CP, Tattersall MHN, eds. New York, Churchill Livingstone, 1992, vol 2, pp 961–970.

21. Price FV, Schwartz PE. Management of ovarian stromal tumors. In *Ovarian Cancer,* Rubin SC, Sutton GP, eds. New York, McGraw-Hill, 1993, pp 405–423, p 410 (21A).

22. Scully RE. Sex cord–stromal tumors. In *Tumors of the Ovary and Maldeveloped Gonads.* Atlas of Tumor Pathology, Second Series, Fascicle 16, Bethesda, Md, Armed Forces Institute of Pathology, 1979, pp 152–214, p 162 (22A), p 163 (22B), p 168 (22C).

# 2

# Pathology
# PART I. PRIMARY OVARIAN EPITHELIAL TUMORS

# 4

# Ovarian Benign Epithelial Tumors

*Liane Deligdisch, M.D.*

## SEROUS CYSTADENOMA AND SEROUS PAPILLARY CYSTADENOMA

Serous cystadenoma and serous papillary cystadenoma are common tumors, representing about 20% of all benign epithelial neoplasms. They are often associated with epithelial inclusion cysts, which are microscopic: both originate from the invagination of the ovarian surface epithelium. These benign tumors are found in women of all ages, from infancy[1] to the late postmenopausal years, but are most prevalent during the reproductive years. They are most commonly unilateral.

### GROSS PATHOLOGY

The ovary appears enlarged because of the presence of a cystic mass that can vary from 1 to over 20 cm. Usually, there is only one cystic cavity (unilocular cysts), but multiple cavities (multilocular cysts) are not uncommon. The fluid is most often clear, "straw" yellow and translucent, and serous. Occasionally, it may be more opaque, mucinous, or blood-tinged. The external surface is generally smooth and may show a vascular pattern or adhesions (Plate 4-1); the internal surface is smooth and glistening in the simple serous cyst, and in the serous papillary cystadenomas shows papillary projections that are white and firm and cover parts, usually not more than one third, of the cystic cavity (Plate 4-2). Papillary structures may be present on the external surface of the cysts.

## MICROSCOPIC APPEARANCE

Papillary structures protruding into the cystic cavity are lined usually by a single layer of epithelial cells resembling the ovarian surface epithelium (Fig. 4-1). The cells are cuboidal, often columnar (Fig. 4-2), displaying various metaplastic cells such as ciliated (Fig. 4-3), mucus-secreting, hobnail (Fig. 4-4), or clear cells. Secretory and ciliated cells tend to occur in patches.[2] The nuclei are round or oval, and regular, with a finely distributed chromatin pattern. Because of the compression by the fluid, the cells can be flattened or low cuboidal (Fig. 4-5). The apical margin of the cytoplasm stains positive for diastase-resistant periodic acid–Schiff (PAS) and mucicarmine because of its mucopolysaccharide content. The underlying connective tissue that represents most of the cystic wall consists of fibroblasts, collagen, and elastic fibers, with interspersed blood vessels. Calcifications are present in about 15% of cases as psammoma bodies, with concentric laminations around a proteinaceous core. In the serous papillary cystadenomas, the connective tissue may form hyalinized, homogenous masses with diffuse calcifications.

## SEROUS CYSTADENOFIBROMA

The serous cystadenofibroma is a variant of the benign serous tumors in which the proliferation of epithelial

**65**

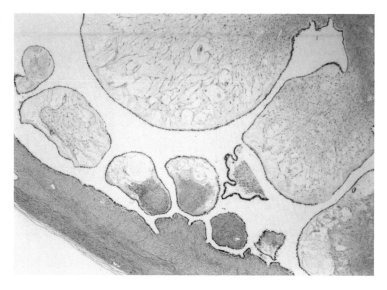

**Fig. 4-1** Serous papillary cystadenoma. Cyst wall (left lower corner) is covered by a layer of epithelial cells and papillations. H&E, ×40.

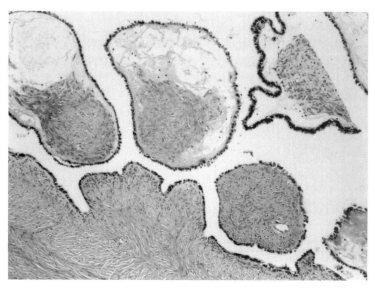

**Fig. 4-2** Same case as Fig. 4-1. Papillary structures with fibroconnective tissue showing edema, lined by a single row of cuboidal epithelial cells resembling ovarian surface epithelium. H&E, ×100.

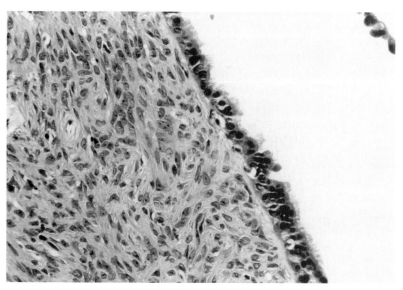

**Fig. 4-3** Serous cystadenoma. Epithelial lining exhibits ciliated cells, similar to fallopian tube lining. H&E, ×250.

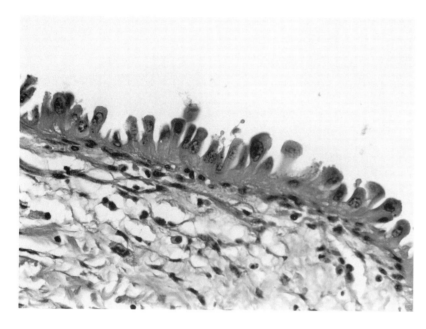

**Fig. 4-4** Serous cystadenoma, showing hobnail cell metaplasia. H&E, ×400.

elements is associated with a proliferation of the ovarian stromal tissue. It is a common tumor, with an age distribution similar to that of the serous cystadenoma.

## GROSS PATHOLOGY

The size ranges from 1 to 20 cm in the largest diameter, with a mean of 9 cm.[3] These tumors are partly cystic and partly solid, the latter component being firm and white (Plate 4-3). The cystic cavities are usually multiple, are of various sizes, and contain a fluid similar to that of the serous cysts. In adenofibroma, the cystic

cavities are small, often only microscopically visible. They are rarely bilateral (8%[3]).

## MICROSCOPIC APPEARANCE

The cyst wall lining is similar to that seen in the serous cystadenomas, with frequent papillary structures and psammoma bodies. The connective tissue is hyalinized, often edematous. Characteristic is a narrow acellular hyalinized layer between the epithelial lining and the connective tissue (Fig. 4-6). Calcifications are often present in the hyalinized stroma.

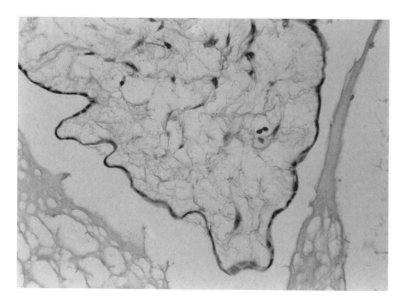

**Fig. 4-5** Serous papillary cystadenoma. Epithelial cells are low cuboidal and flat. H&E, ×100.

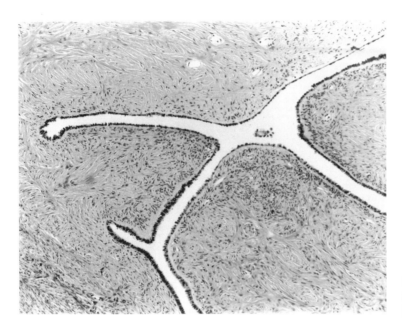

**Fig. 4-6** Serous cystadenofibroma. Note the narrow acellular hyalinized layer between the epithelial lining and the connective tissue. H&E, ×100.

## SEROUS ADENOFIBROMAS

Serous adenofibromas are less common and appear as solid tumors similar to the ovarian fibromas. The glandular spaces are lined by epithelium similar to that seen in the serous tumors (Figs. 4-7 and 4-8). The stroma ranges from cellular in the zones surrounding the glands to hyalinized and acellular.

Cellular crowding, atypia, nuclear pleomorphism, and mitotic activity are not present in the above-described entities.

## MUCINOUS CYSTADENOMAS

Mucinous cystadenomas constitute about 20% of all benign ovarian neoplasms. It is generally accepted that they are of epithelial origin, originating in mucinous metaplasia of the ovarian surface epithelium, because of their frequent association with serous and endometriotic tumors. Endodermal differentiation of a benign cystic teratoma has been postulated in their histogenesis because of their association with cystic teratoma in 5% of cases[4] and because of the presence of goblet and argen-

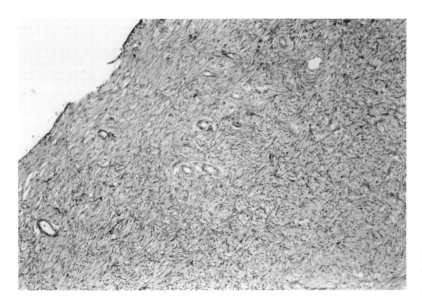

**Fig. 4-7** Serous adenofibroma (low power) composed of densely fibrotic connective tissue and tubular epithelial structures. H&E, ×40.

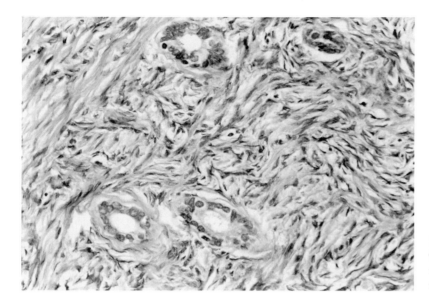

**Fig. 4-8** Serous adenofibroma (high power). Cuboidal and ciliated epithelium lines tubular structures embedded in dense connective tissue. H&E, × 250.

taffin cells. This tumor occurs mostly in young women but can be seen at any age, with the highest frequency between the third and the fifth decade. It is occasionally diagnosed in pregnant women, sometimes associated with luteinization of the adjacent stroma.[5]

## GROSS APPEARANCE

The cystic tumors are multilocular and may reach very large sizes, up to 50 cm in greatest diameter (Plates 4-4 and 4-5). In fact, some of the largest human tumors are ovarian mucinous neoplasms. Multiple bluish cysts are bulging on the external surface. The content of these cysts is an opaque, sticky, stringy material, whitish to bluish, exuding from multiple cystic cavities of various sizes. Areas that may feel solid on palpation turn out to be composed of multiple small cysts with a honeycomb structure on cut section. Because of their large size and common association with pregnancy, these tumors may present with torsion.

## MICROSCOPIC APPEARANCE

The cystic cavities are lined by a single layer of tall, columnar cells, with basally located nuclei and a mucus-filled cytoplasm. The uniformity of the lining cells is characteristic (Figs. 4-9 and 4-10). The underlying stromal tissue is generally less developed than in the serous tumors and may contain occasional calcifications. Two types of mucinous cells can be identified: endocervical and gastrointestinal types, the latter including goblet cells and argentaffin or argyrophil neuroendocrine cells (Fig. 4-11). The mucinous content of the cells is a glycoprotein, containing intestinal mucin.[6] At the periphery of some cystic cavities numerous benign mucinous tumors display small cavities or "daughter cysts"[2] lined by epithelial cells with signs of activity, consisting of hyperchromatic nuclei and mitotic activity (Fig. 4-12). More complex patterns, piling up, and tufting of the epithelium with atypia characterize tumors of borderline malignancy and are described separately. The epithelium may be cuboidal or flat because of the compression by mucus, which may leak into the surrounding stroma (Fig. 4-13) and elicit inflammatory or foreign body reaction. This lesion is called pseudomyxoma ovarii.

Mucinous tumors are often associated with other tumors of epithelial derivation, such as serous or endometrioid, or with sex cord–derived structures.[7] There have been reports of associated osteoclastomas[8] and carcinoids.[9,10]

Mucinous tumors can also be associated with Peutz-Jeghers syndrome along with cervical adenoma malignum and ovarian sex cord tumors.[11]

## ENDOMETRIOID TUMORS

Benign endometrioid neoplasms of the ovary resemble proliferative or inactive endometrium. Endometriosis of the ovary is not considered to be a tumor by most authors and is not included in the World Health Organization (WHO) classification of 1973. Endometrioid

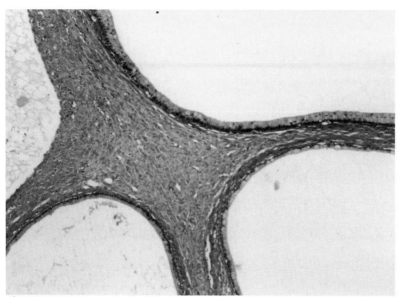

**Fig. 4-9**

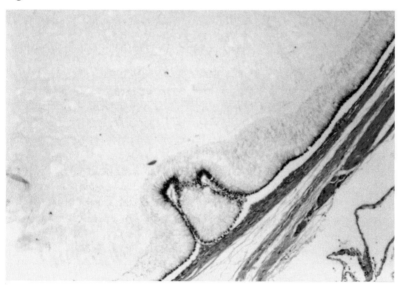

**Fig. 4-10**

**Figs. 4-9 and 4-10** Mucinous cystadenoma, showing columnar cells with mucus in the apical portion of the cytoplasm and regular basal nuclei. Stromal septa separate cystic cavities. H&E, ×100.

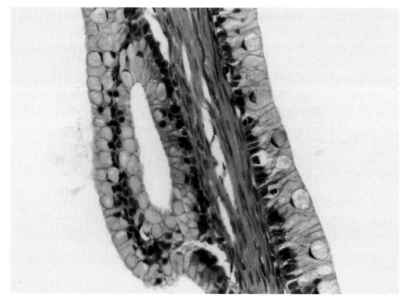

**Fig. 4-11** Goblet cells are found in the lining of mucinous cystadenoma. H&E, ×400.

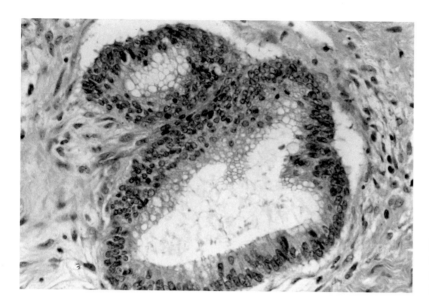

**Fig. 4-12** Proliferating, active "daughter cysts" displaying hyperchromatic nuclei and mitotic activity at the bottom of the crypts. H&E, ×400.

cystadenofibroma is an accepted entity and is also designated as proliferative endometrioid tumor (PET).[12] Atypical endometriosis has been described to be associated with ovarian neoplasms.[13] Despite some overlapping, the risk factors for benign serous and mucinous tumors are different from those of endometrioid tumors.[14]

## GROSS APPEARANCE

Benign endometrioid tumors are cystic structures of various sizes, averaging 10 cm in diameter, with a fibrous wall, which often displays brownish discoloration. The surface is generally smooth. On cut section, the single or multiple cystic cavities contain clear yellowish fluid (Plate 4-6).

## MICROSCOPIC APPEARANCE

Endometrioid adenofibromas, or PETs, display branching tubular glands, lined by columnar epithelium resembling that of endometrial glands. Small solid aggregates of epithelial cells can be identified.[12] Mitoses are uncommon; squamous metaplasia is often present. The stroma, unlike that in nonneoplastic endometriosis, is mostly fibrotic (Fig. 4-14). With rare exceptions, no cyclic endometrial changes are noted.

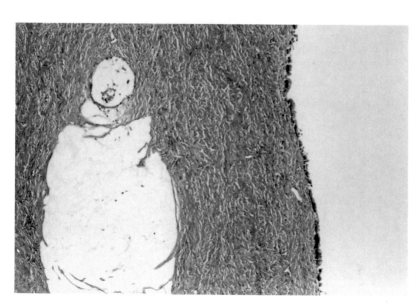

**Fig. 4-13** Mucinous cystadenoma, showing cystic lining (right) and mucus "leaking" into the surrounding stroma. H&E, ×40.

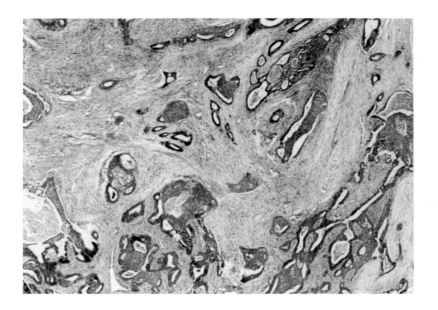

**Fig. 4-14** Endometrioid adenofibroma, showing branching endometrial-type tubular glands with squamous metaplasia. Stroma is dense fibrotic, unlike that seen in endometriosis. H&E, ×100.

An uncommon variant of benign endometrioid tumors in the ovary is the adenomyoma, in which the smooth muscle component may arise in the endometrioid stroma.[15]

## BRENNER TUMORS

Brenner tumors appear to originate from the surface epithelium of the ovary, which undergoes metaplasia to urothelial-type nests, similar to the Walthard's nests. The epithelial (versus mesonephric) nature of this tumor is supported by the frequent association with other müllerian epithelial elements (mucinous, serous). Brenner tumors are often a microscopic incidental finding. Their peak incidence is in the fifth decade, and bilaterality is found in about 6 to 7%. Antigenic and ultrastructural characteristics show similarities to the urothelium.[16,17] Argyrophil cells were identified in 39% of Brenner tumors.[17]

### GROSS PATHOLOGY

Most tumors are small, less than 2 cm in diameter; few exceed 10 cm. There are firm, solid, well-circumscribed, white-yellowish, and rarely cystic. (Plate 4-7).

#### Microscopic Appearance

Epithelial nests composed of urothelial-type cells are scattered in a dense cellular ovarian stroma. The cells are polygonal or oval, with well-defined margins, round nuclei often exhibiting a longitudinal grooving ("coffee bean" appearance). This feature is not constant and not as characteristic as it is for granulosa cell tumors. These nests often show microcystic cavities with a mucinous eosinophilic acellular content, lined by mucin-secreting metaplastic cells. The stroma resembles that in adenofibromas, often with calcifications (Figs. 4-15 and 4-16). Occasional luteinization of the stroma has been observed.

## PROLIFERATING VARIANTS OF BENIGN EPITHELIAL OVARIAN TUMORS

Cellular crowding, piling up of epithelium, loss of polarity, increased nuclear cytoplasmic ratio, and mitotic activity may occur in all of the above described tumors. Probably the most commonly seen proliferating variant is that found in the mucinous cystadenoma, in which the marked increase in nuclear size is obviously due to a high proliferating activity that is benign, since even the very large mucinous cystadenomas do not metastasize.

The natural history of benign proliferating tumors is different from that of borderline epithelial tumors or tumors of low malignant potential (LMP), while the histologic features are often overlapping. Criteria to differentiate between the two are not always unanimous.[12,17,18] Some helpful hints are summarized in Table 4-1.

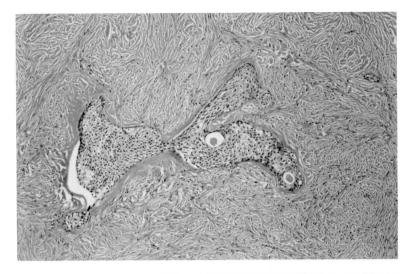

**Fig. 4-15** Brenner tumor, nest of transitional epithelium with small cystic cavities surrounded by dense fibrous tissue. H&E, ×100.

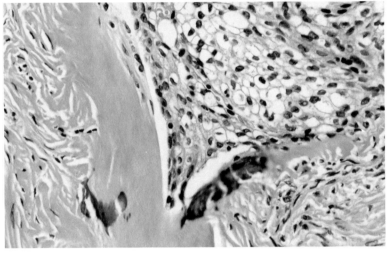

**Fig. 4-16** Brenner tumor, transitional epithelium with nuclei displaying focal central grooving. Stroma is hyalinized and calcified. H&E, ×400.

**Table 4-1**   Proliferating Benign vs. Borderline (LMP) Ovarian Tumors

|  | *Proliferating Benign Epithelial Tumors* | *Borderline (LMP) Tumors* |
|---|---|---|
| Serous cystadenoma | Pseudostratification with tubal-type, ciliated, or secretory cells, resulting uneven apical border | True stratification of epithelium |
|  | No detached clusters of epithelial cells | Epithelial budding and tufting |
|  | Complex papillary pattern with no atypia | Detached clusters of epithelial cells |
|  | Few or no mitoses | Nuclear atypia: prominent nucleoli, hyperchromasia |
|  |  | Mitotic activity up to 4/10 hpf |
| Mucinous cystadenoma | Endocervical and colonic type epithelium about equal | Predominance of colonic over endocervical epithelium |
|  | Pseudostratification, some hyperchromatic nuclei, less mucus content in cells | True stratification, hyperchromatic nuclei, prominent nucleoli, less mucus content in cells |
|  | "Daughter cysts" at the periphery of the cystic cavities | Gland formation and filigree pattern |
| Endometrioid tumors (endometrioid cystadenofibroma) | Glandular, crowding, complex pattern, occasional mitoses, squamous metaplasia | Closely packed glands, cribriform pattern in epithelial islands embedded in fibrous stroma, without invasion |
| Brenner tumor | Small, mostly solid tumors | Grossly large, cystic tumors* |
|  | Transitional epithelium hyperplasia | Papillary structures |
|  | Mild nuclear atypia, no mitoses | Mild nuclear atypia, few mitoses |

*Because of the small number of cases and conflicting opinions, definitive criteria for the differential diagnosis between proliferating and borderline Brenner tumor are not yet established.

## PLATES

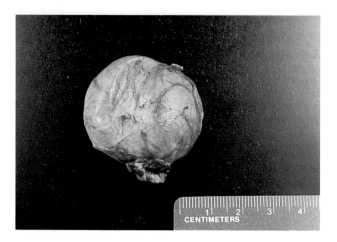

**Plate 4-1** Serous cystadenoma. External surface is smooth, showing vascularity and some adhesions.

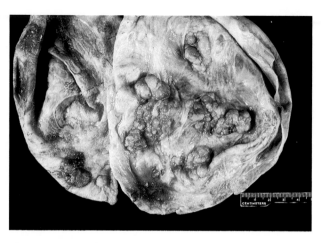

**Plate 4-2** Internal surface of papillary serous cystadenoma with papillary projections into the cystic cavity.

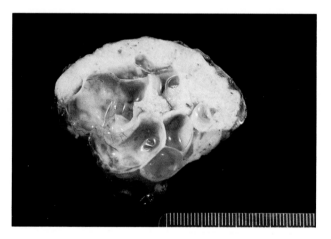

**Plate 4-3** Ovarian cystadenofibroma with cystic and solid portions.

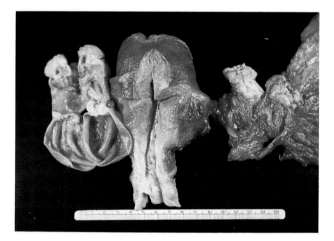

**Plate 4-4** Endometrioid cystadenofibroma, left ovary. Adenofibroma, right ovary.

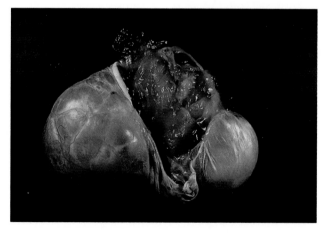

**Plate 4-5** Mucinous cystadenoma. External surface is smooth, cavity filled by a gelatinous material.

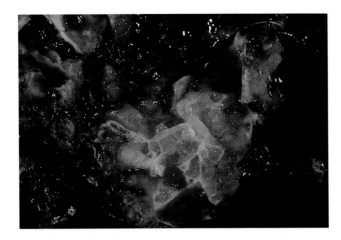

**Plate 4-6** Mucinous cystadenoma showing multilocular cystic structure. A microscopic benign teratoma was found.

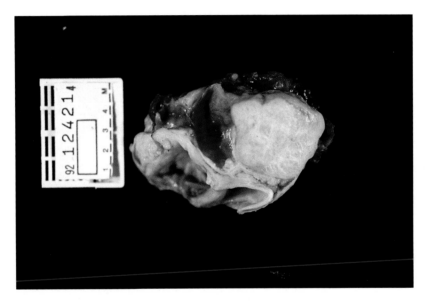

**Plate 4-7** Brenner's tumor

## REFERENCES

1. Moore JG, Schiffrin BS, Erez S. Ovarian tumors in infancy, childhood and adolescence. *Am J Obstet Gynecol* 93:850–866, 1965.
2. Russel P, Bannatyne P. *Surgical Pathology of the Ovaries.* Serous tumours. Edinburgh, Churchill Livingstone, 1989, p 200.
3. Czernobilsky B. In *Blaustein's Pathology of the Female Genital Tract,* 3d ed. Kurman R, ed. New York Springer-Verlag, 1987, p 568.
4. Cariker M, Dockerty MB. Mucinous cystadenoma and mucinous cystadenocarcinomas of the ovary: A clinical pathologic study of 355 cases. *Cancer* 7:302–310, 1954.
5. Pascal RR, Grecco LA. Mucinous cystadenoma with stromal luteinization and hilar cell hyperplasia during pregnancy. *Hum Pathol* 19:179–180, 1988.
6. Fenoglio CM, Cottral GA, Ferenczy A, Richart RM. Mucinous tumors of the ovary: III. Histochemical studies. *Gynecol Oncol* 4:151–157, 1976.
7. Roth LM, Clear R, Rosenfield RL. Sertoli–Leydig cell tumor of the ovary with an associated mucinous cystadenoma: An ultrastructural and endocrine study. *Lab Invest* 31:648–657, 1974.
8. Lorentzen M. Giant cell tumor of the ovary. *Virchows Arch* A 388:113–122, 1980.
9. Alenghat E, Okagaki T, Talerman A. Primary carcinoid tumor of the ovary. *Cancer* 58:777–783, 1986.
10. Waxman M, Damjanovi, Alpert L, Sardinsky T. Composite mucinous ovarian neoplasms associated with Sertoli–Leydig and carcinoid tumors. *Cancer* 47:2044–2052, 1981.
11. Chen KT. Female genital tract tumors in Peutz-Jeghers syndrome. *Hum Pathol* 17:858–861, 1986.
12. Snyder RR, Norris HJ, Tavassoli T. Endometrioid proliferative and low malignant potential tumors of the ovary. A clinico-pathologic study of 46 cases. *Am J Surg Pathol* 12:661–671, 1988.
13. Le Grenade AM, Silverberg SG. Ovarian tumors associated with atypical endometriosis. *Hum Pathol* 19:1080–1084, 1988.
14. Parazzini F, La Vecchia C, Franceschi S, Negri E, Cecchetti G. Risk factors for endometrioid, mucinous and serous benign ovarian cysts. *Int J Epidemiol* 18:108–112, 1989.
15. McDougal RA, Roth LM. Ovarian adenomyoma associated with an endometriotic cyst. *South Med J* 79:640–642, 1986.
16. Santini D, Gelli MC, Mazzoleni G, et al. Brenner tumor of the ovary: A correlative histologic histochemical immunohistochemical and ultrastructural investigation. *Hum Pathol* 20:787–795, 1989.
17. Aguiree P, Scully RE, Wolfe HJ, De Lellis RA. Argyrophil cells in Brenner tumors: Histochemical and immunohistochemical analysis. *Int J Gynecol Pathol* 5:223–234, 1986.
18. Roth LM, Dallenbach-Hellweg G, Czernobilsky B. Ovarian Brenner tumors: I. metaplastic, proliferating and of low malignant potential. *Cancer* 56:582–591, 1985.

# 5

# Epithelial Ovarian Tumors of Low Malignant Potential (Borderline)

*Liane Deligdisch, M.D.*

Ovarian tumors of low malignant potential (LMP) were incorporated in the WHO histologic classification of ovarian tumors in 1964. Their histologic characteristics and natural history are different from those of invasive serous carcinoma. LMP serous tumors should not be considered a transition stage between benign and malignant tumors, although they may include a spectrum of changes reflecting various degrees of severity. These tumors often recur, sometimes as late as 15 years after the initial diagnosis, spreading to the peritoneum without invading. Their histologic appearance is identical in the recurrences to that of the primary tumors.[1] Synonymous terms such as *tumors with atypical proliferation,*[2] *borderline malignancy,*[3] or *intraepithelial neoplasia*[4] designate changes that include cellular proliferation with no destructive invasion of the ovarian stroma. The LMP tumors occur in younger patients, and the survival rates of such patients are significantly better than those of patients with invasive carcinomas.[5-8] Table 5-1 summarizes the criteria for differentials up between LMP and invasive ovarian tumors.

## SEROUS PAPILLARY CARCINOMA OF LMP

Serous papillary carcinomas of LMP are the most common LMP tumors,[1,9] representing about 15% of all serous papillary carcinomas. There are no characteristic gross changes to distinguish these tumors from serous papillary cystadenomas (Plate 5-1). More abundant papillary components may occasionally cover the cyst wall. Extensive sampling of the more solid components of the tumor is recommended, about 1 section per 1 to 2 cm of tumor. Up to 40% of LMP ovarian tumors are unilateral.[10] Morphometric studies have contributed valuable discriminating criteria to identify the LMP tumors.[11-14] The microscopic characteristics consist of changes in architecture, cytologic appearance, and proliferative pattern. There is epithelial budding of the papillary structures creating filigree patterns and a tendency of cell clusters to detach into the cystic space (Figs. 5-1 to 5-3). The piling up of epithelial cells (Fig. 5-4) may reach up to nine layers.[3] Cytologically, the nuclear area and the nuclear/cytoplasmic ratio are increased (Fig. 5-5). Nucleoli and chromatin pattern are prominent (Fig. 5-6). Nuclear atypia in tumors of LMP is not extremely severe, and acceptable mitotic activity is up to 2 per 10 high-power fields. Characteristically, there is no stromal invasion and the stroma is composed of mature connective tissue. Psammoma bodies are frequently present. Microinvasion is a controversial issue: it represents perhaps the early stage of an invasive cancer rather than a borderline tumor (Fig. 5-7). The stromal reaction accompanying invasion consists of a loose ground substance and an inflammatory, mostly round cell, infiltrate, absent in some reported cases of microinvasion.[15] Recurrent LMP tumors have a similar histo-

**Table 5-1** Borderline (LMP) vs. Invasive Ovarian Epithelial Tumors

| | Borderline (LMP) Tumors | Invasive Tumors |
|---|---|---|
| Peritoneal lesions | Uncommon | Frequent |
| Bilaterality | Less frequent | Frequent |
| Peak age | 45 years | 65 years |
| Gross papillations | Mostly intracystic | May fill cavity; seen on surface |
| Necrosis, hemorrhage | Rare | Frequent |
| Nuclear atypia | Mild to moderate | Severe |
| Giant and bizarre cells | Absent | Frequent |
| Mitotic activity | Less than 4/10 hpf (more in mucinous tumors) | High |
| Stroma | Dense, mature | Loose, immature |
| Invasion of stroma | Absent | Present |
| Stroma reaction | Absent | Present |

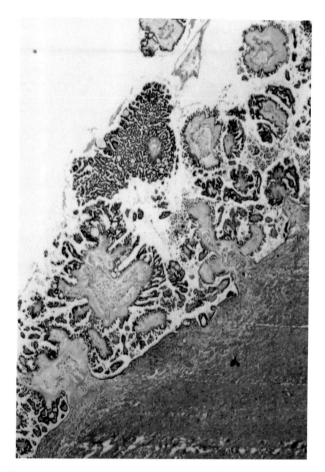

**Fig. 5-2** Ovarian tumor of LMP, showing florid papillary proliferation with filigree pattern. Stromal invasion is absent. H&E, × 40.

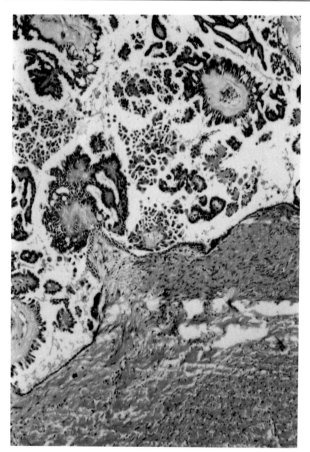

**Fig. 5-1** Ovarian tumor of LMP, showing papillary projections with abundant epithelial proliferation and numerous detached clusters. There is no invasion of the dense, mature, ovarian stroma. H&E, × 100.

logic appearance to that of the primary tumors (Fig. 5-8). About 15% of serous papillary LMP tumors are associated with peritoneal spread and represent stage III lesions. The peritoneal "implants" are usually similar to the ovarian lesions and are seen on the serosal surface or in the fibrofatty tissue, often in the proximity of psammoma bodies (Fig. 5-9). The prognosis of stage III LMP ovarian tumors in terms of recurrence and persistence is less favorable.[1] LMP ovarian cystadenofibromas are diagnosed according to the same criteria as their pure serous counterparts (Fig. 5-10).

## MUCINOUS TUMORS OF LMP

The incidence of mucinous tumors of LMP is about 13% and varies in different reports.[1,16] As is true of their serous counterparts, there is no characteristic gross difference from the benign mucinous ovarian tumors;

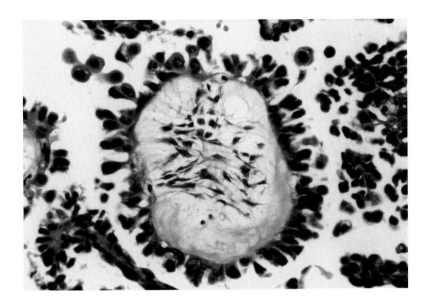

**Fig. 5-3** Ovarian tumor of LMP: marked epithelial proliferation and detached individual cells and cell clusters. H&E, ×400.

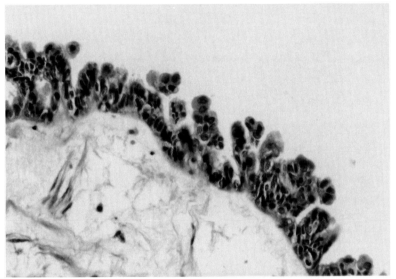

**Fig. 5-4** Ovarian tumor of LMP: proliferation of epithelial cells with piling up of the layers and small detached cell clusters. H&E, ×200.

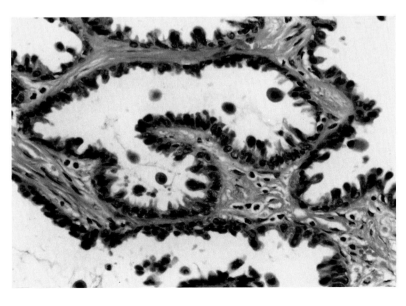

**Fig. 5-5** Ovarian tumor of LMP: mild to moderate nuclear atypia and increased nuclear/cytoplasmic ratio, especially in detached epithelial cells. H&E, ×100.

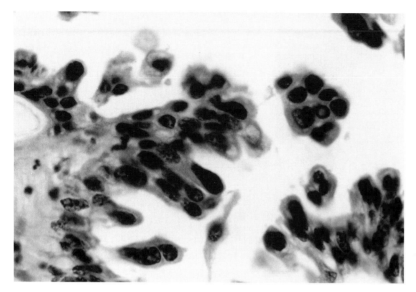

**Fig. 5-6** Ovarian tumor of LMP: moderate nuclear atypia, hyperchromasia, and coarse chromatin pattern. H&E, ×500.

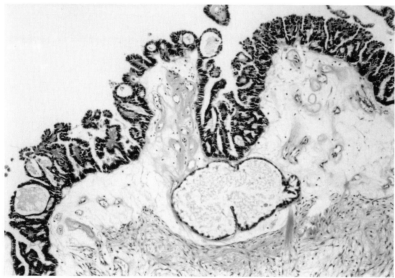

**Fig. 5-7** Questionable microinvasion. Stroma is loose around invaginated epithelial structure, but no inflammatory infiltrate is seen. H&E, ×100.

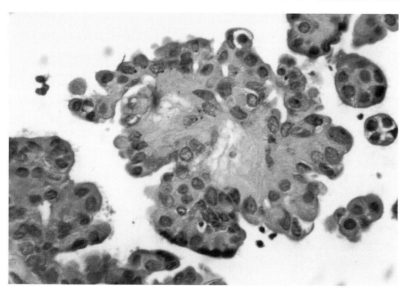

**Fig. 5-8** Papillary structure in recurrent LMP ovarian tumor, histologically similar to that diagnosed 15 years before. H&E, ×400.

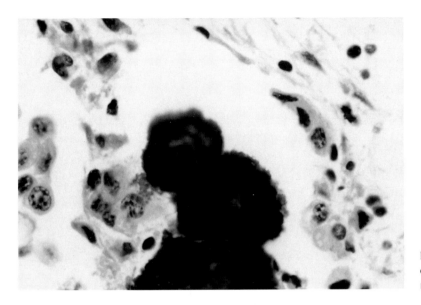

**Fig. 5-9** Psammoma bodies and papillary proliferation of peritoneal surface in LMP ovarian tumor. H&E, ×400.

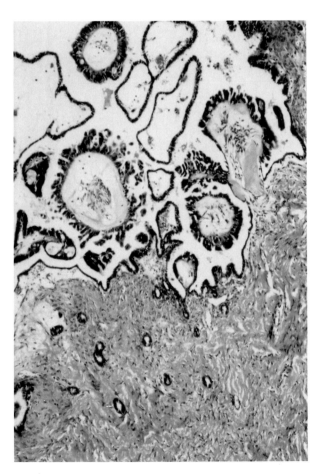

**Fig. 5-10** Adenofibroma and LMP tumor. H&E, ×100.

the lesion is often found in areas of thickening and honeycombing of the subcapsular region (Plate 5-2).

Microscopically, this tumor is less well defined than its serous counterpart, and the diagnosis is more difficult. Piling up of epithelial cells and glandular crowding with a filigree pattern are the architectural changes (Fig. 5-11). The individual cells show a decrease in mucin content in the cytoplasm, a higher nuclear/cytoplasmic ratio, nuclear membrane infoldings, and higher mitotic activity than that acceptable for the serous LMP tumors (Fig. 5-12). Mitotic activity is predominant at the periphery of mucinous locules in which small acini lined by cells with hyperchromatic enlarged nuclei and diminished cytoplasmic mucin content are seen. They seem to grow in a centrifugal manner, but invasion of the stroma is difficult to assess (Fig. 5-13). Glandular tufts and papillary structures with less connective tissue than in the serous tumors are common (Fig. 5-14). Numerous goblet cells can be seen, as in a colonic-type mucosa. Mixed mucinous-serous ovarian tumors of LMP (Fig. 5-15) are not uncommon.

An interesting, though rarely documented, finding is the hyerplasia of fallopian tube epithelium associated with LMP ovarian tumors, as a possible example of "field effect."[17]

## ENDOMETRIOID LMP TUMORS

This subtype has been described relatively recently and is still controversial.[3,10,16,18,19] Grossly, the tumors resemble the benign cystadenofibromas (Plate 5-3). Microscopically, the endometrial-like epithelium prolifer-

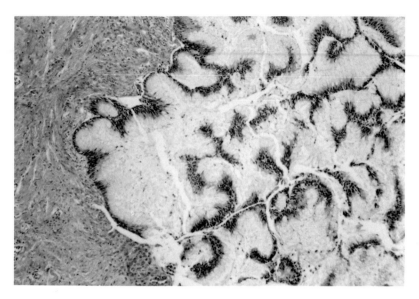

**Fig. 5-11** Mucinous tumor of LMP. Note marked glandular crowding. H&E, ×100.

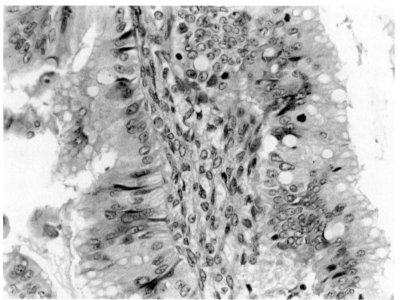

**Fig. 5-12** Mucinous tumor of LMP. Epithelial cells show piling up higher nuclear/cytoplasmic ratios, nuclear infoldings, and reduced mucin secretion, as well as mitoses. H&E, ×400.

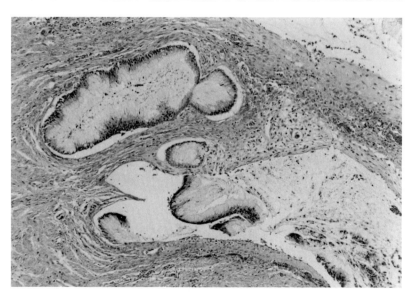

**Fig. 5-13** Mucinous tumor of LMP. Stromal invasion is difficult to assess. Edema and inflammatory infiltrates (right) may represent reaction to mucin "leaks." H&E, ×100.

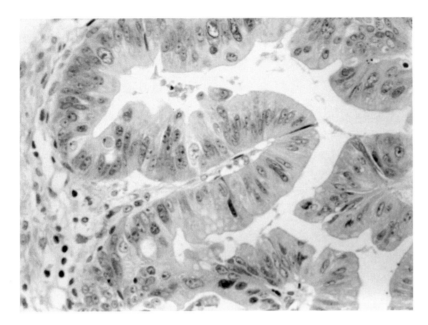

**Fig. 5-14** Mucinous tumor of LMP showing glandular tufts, moderate nuclear atypia, and diminished mucin secretion. H&E, ×400.

ates in a fashion similar to that seen in the endometrial hyperplasia, with solid nests of squamoid morules in up to 50% of the cases and atypical features (Fig. 5-16) such as tufting, bridging, and epithelial stratification.[16,18] Papillary proliferation may also be present as well as cellular atypia reminiscent of that seen in atypical endometrial hyperplasia with an occasional cribriform pattern. The adjacent stroma is mature, and the lining may show squamous metaplasia. In invasive endometrioid carcinoma, one finds stromal edema and inflammatory infiltrates.[2]

Endometrioid tumors of LMP were also described

without an adenofibromatous pattern and associated with microinvasion.[19]

## CLEAR CELL CARCINOMA OF LMP

Clear cell carcinoma of LMP is an unusual variant of an adenofibromatous tumor in which cords and tubules of atypical clear cells are noted, displaying mitotic activity up to 3 per 10 high-power fields[2] but no invasion of the stroma.[16,19,20] They often occur in association with

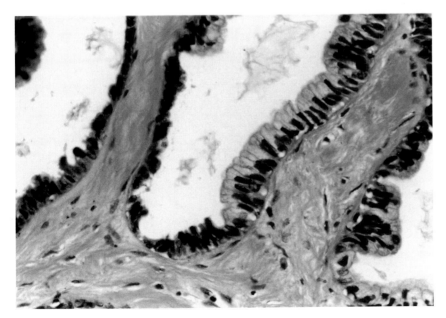

**Fig. 5-15** Mixed mucinous and serous tumor of LMP, with tufting and mild atypia of epithelium. H&E, ×400.

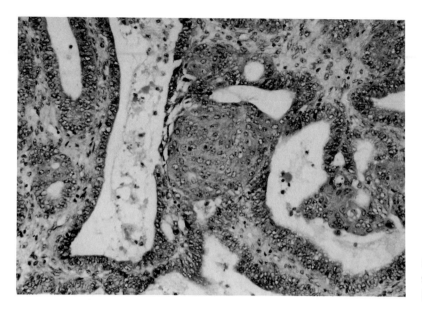

**Fig. 5-16** Endometrioid tumor of LMP. Note similarity to endometrial adenomatous hyperplasia and squamoid morule. H&E, ×200.

endometriosis.[2] Grossly, they may display a honeycombed structure with minute cysts or may present as a cystadenofibroma with smooth capsular surface, sometime reaching a large size (up to 23 cm in diameter).

## BRENNER TUMORS OF LMP

These tumors are difficult to define. They are rare, and their microscopic configuration is somewhat intermediate between that of benign proliferating and malignant Brenner tumors.[21,22] The epithelial proliferation may exhibit, in addition to the typical urothelial type nests, papillary structures with coarse connective tissue, and cysts lined by multilayered atypical epithelium, some reminiscent of low-grade transitional epithelium of the urinary bladder with mucin-secreting, ciliated, and squamous metaplastic cells in variable amounts.

Proliferative variants of benign epithelial tumors should be distinguished from the tumors of low malignant potential because of their different biologic behavior and management. Histologically, this is not always possible because of overlapping features. A number of criteria are proposed,[23,24] but further studies of DNA ploidy, tumor markers, and morphometry may contribute to a better understanding of the biologic significance of histologic characteristics.

# PLATES

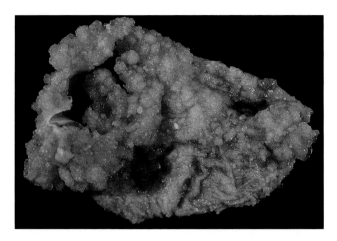

**Plate 5-1** Serous papillary tumor of LMP. Numerous papillary excrescences protrude into the cystic cavity.

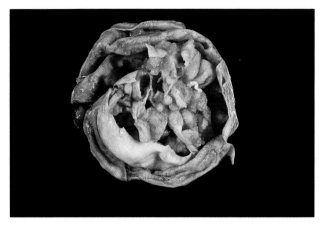

**Plate 5-2** Mucinous tumor of LMP. The more advanced histologic lesions were found in the central honeycomb region.

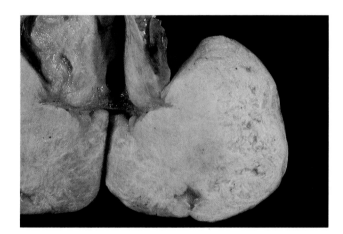

**Plate 5-3** Ovarian adenofibroma with endometrioid tumor of LMP.

# REFERENCES

1. Bostwick DG, Tazelaar HD, Ballon SC, Hendrickson MR, Kempson RL. Ovarian epithelial tumors of borderline malignancy. A clinical and pathologic study of 109 cases. *Cancer* 58:2052–2065, 1986.

2. Russell P, Ballantyne P. Surgical Pathology of the Ovaries. Edinburgh, Churchill Livingstone, 1989, p 191–192.

3. Serov SF, Scully RE, Sobin LH. *Histological Typing of Ovarian Tumors.* International Histological Classification of Tumors, no. 9. Geneva, World Health Organization, 1973, p 37 (3a), pp 17–18 (3b).

4. Yoonessi M, Crickard K, Celik C. Yoonessi S. Borderline epithelial tumors of the ovary: Ovarian intraepithelial neoplasia. *Obstet Gynecol Surv* 43:435–444, 1988.

5. Gallup DG, Cody WM, Metheny WP, Talledoo E. Epithelial tumors of the ovary in women less than 40 years old. *South Med J* 81:10–14, 1988.

6. Chien RT, Rettenmaier Ma, Micha JP, DiSaia PJ. Ovarian epithelial tumors of low malignant potential. *Surg Gynecol Obstet* 169:143–146, 1989.

7. Bernhill D, Heller P, Brzozowski P, Advani H, Gallup D, Park R. Epithelial ovarian carcinoma of low malignant potential. *Obstet Gynecol* 65:53–59, 1985.

8. Harlow BL, Weiss NS, Lefton S. Epidemiology of borderline ovarian tumors. *J Natl Cancer Inst* 78:71–74, 1987.

9. England MJ, Sonnendecker EW, Margolius KA. Epithelial tumors of low malignant potential. *SA Fr Med J* 70:343–348, 1986.

10. Czernobilsky B. Common epithelial tumors of the ovary. In *Blaustein's Pathology of the Female Genital Tract.* 3d ed, Kurman R, ed. New York, Springer-Verlag, p. 578.

11. Baak JP, Fox H, Langley FA, Buckley CH. The prognostic value of morphometry in ovarian epithelial tumors of borderline malignancy. *Int J Gynecol Pathol* 4:186–191, 1985.

12. Komitowski D, Janson C, Szamaborski J, Czernobilski B. Quantitative nuclear morphology in the diagnosis of ovarian tumors of low malignant potential (borderline). *Cancer* 64:905–910, 1989.

13. Hytiroglou P, Harpaz N, Heller D, Lin Z, Deligdisch L, Gil J. Differential diagnosis of borderline and invasive serous cystadenocarcinomas of the ovary by computerized interactive morphometry of nuclear features. *Cancer* 69:988–992, 1992.

14. Baak JP, Chan KK, Stolk JG, Kenemans P. Prognostic factors in borderline and invasive ovarian tumors of the common epithelial type. *Pathol Res Pract* 182:755–774, 1987.

15. Bell DA, Scully RE. Ovarian serous borderline tumors with stromal microinvasion: A report of 21 cases. *Hum Pathol* 21:397–403, 1990.

16. Kao GF, Norris HJ. Unusual cystadenofribroma: Endometrioid, mucinous and clear cell types. *Obstet Gynecol* 54:729–736, 1979.

17. Robey SS, Silva EG. Epithelial hyperplasia of the fallopian tube. Its association with borderline tumors of the ovary. *Int J Gynecol Pathol* 8:214–220, 1989.

18. Bell DA, Scully RE. Benign and borderline clear cell adenofibroma of the ovary. *Cancer* 56:2922, 2931, 1985.

19. Roth LM, Langley FA, Fox H, Wheeler JE, Czernobilsky B. Ovarian clear cell adenofibromatous tumors: Benign of low malignant potential and associated with invasive clear cell carcinoma. *Cancer* 53:1156, 1163, 1984.

20. Bell DA, Scully RE. Atypical and borderline endometrioid adenofibromas of the ovary. A report of 27 cases. *Am J Surg Pathol* 9:205–214, 1985.

21. Trebeck CE, Friedlander ML, Russell P, Baird PJ. Brenner tumors of the ovary: A study of the histology, immunohistochemistry and cellular DNA content in benign, borderline and malignant ovarian tumors. *Pathology* 19:241–246, 1987.

22. Roth LM, Dallenbach-Hellweg G, Czernobilsky B. Ovarian Brenner tumors: I. Metaplastic, proliferating and of low malignant potential. *Cancer* 56:582–591, 1985.

23. Ulbright TM, Roth LM. Common epithelial tumors of the ovary: Proliferating and of low malignant potential. *Semin Diagn Pathol* 2:2–15, 1985.

24. Carter J, Atkinson K, Coppleson M, et al. A comparative study of proliferative (borderline) and invasive epithelial tumors in young women. *Aust NZ J Obstet Gynaecol* 29:245–249, 1989.

# 6

# Ovarian Malignant Epithelial Tumors

*Liane Deligdisch, M.D.*

COMMON TUMORS:
Serous papillary cystadenocarcinoma
Serous papillary peritoneal carcinoma
Mucinous cystadenocarcinoma
Endometrioid adenocarcinoma
Clear cell carcinoma

UNCOMMON TUMORS:
Malignant mixed mesodermal tumors
Small cell carcinoma
Malignant Brenner and transitional cell carcinoma
Undifferentiated carcinoma

The epithelial malignant tumors of the ovary represent almost 90% of all ovarian malignancies. The high mortality of patients with these tumors is because the great majority are diagnosed in stage III or IV, when the ovarian tumors have spread to the peritoneal cavity. They originate from the surface epithelium of the ovary, which is an extension of the primitive coelomic mesothelium. During the embryonal development, the latter invaginates laterally, giving rise to the müllerian ducts. The heterogenous histologic patterns of the ovarian epithelial tumors are reminiscent of various portions of the müllerian duct—derived structures: the serous tumors of the fallopian tube, the mucinous tumors of the endocervical glands, and the endometrioid tumors of the uterine epithelium. The epithelial tumors of the ovaries, therefore, are analogous to endometrial, endocervical, and (rare) fallopian tube epithelial tumors. Clear cell, mixed mesodermal, small cell, and transi-

tional cell carcinomas are uncommon and may occur in the ovary or in portions of the müllerian ducts with a similar histologic appearance.

Coexistent histologic patterns of various epithelial types are common in this group of tumors and are designated as mixed epithelial tumors.

## SEROUS PAPILLARY CYSTADENOCARCINOMA

Serous papillary cystadenocarcinoma is the most frequent ovarian cancer: about 1% of all women develop this cancer, mostly after the age of 40. More than one-half of serous papillary adenocarcinomas are bilateral, and by the time of diagnosis, most are associated with peritoneal, especially omental, spread. The metastatic involvement may be more voluminous than the primary ovarian tumors. Metastases from one ovary to the other are common, supported by the finding of tumor cells in the lymphatics. Whether the contralateral ovary is the site of a second primary or of a metastatic involvement is rather of academic interest.

### GROSS PATHOLOGY

The size of the ovarian tumor may vary from a few centimeters to over 30 cm in greatest diameter. The

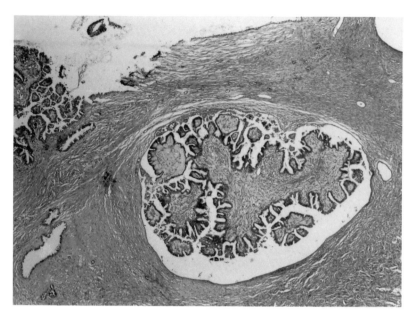

**Fig. 6-1** Ovarian well-differentiated serous (grade 1) papillary carcinoma growing on the surface (left upper corner) and into cystic cavities in the ovarian parenchyma. H&E, ×100.

tumors are usually cystic. Papillary excrescences are seen on cut section, protruding into the cystic cavity and often on the surface of the ovary. The consistency is firm with softened areas in the larger tumors, representing necrosis. The color is whitish-gray or tan and rarely hemorrhagic (Plates 6-1 to 6-3). There are often adhesions to the adjacent structures, fallopian tubes, omentum, and broad ligaments. The tumor may represent a large mass in which the ovarian structure becomes unrecognizable.

## MICROSCOPIC APPEARANCE

The predominant features are papillary structures composed of a fibrovascular stalk that may range from irregular coarse to slender and delicate, covered by neoplastic epithelial cells. The degree of differentiation is related to the proportion between epithelial and connective tissue (the more epithelium, the less the differentiation) and to the cellular atypia. Well-differentiated serous papillary adenocarcinomas (grade 1) have a well-represented papillary component, with more abundant connective tissue (Figs. 6-1 to 6-3). Moderately differentiated tumors (grade 2) show solid areas of malignant epithelial cells with less well formed connective tissue stalks (Figs. 6-4 to 6-7), and poorly differentiated tumors (grade 3) consist mostly of solid sheets of epithelial tumor cells with occasional papillary structures. The coalescing epithelial papillae may form clefts with a glandlike appearance (Fig. 6-8): these are not real adenocarcinomas as seen in endometrioid carcinomas, although transitional forms between the two are not uncommon (Fig. 6-9). Nuclear pleomorphism is common, and bizarre multinucleated giant cells are seen in the less differentiated tumors (Figs. 6-10 to 6-12). Psammoma bodies are concentrically laminated calcified structures, associated with approximately one-third of the serous papillary ovarian carcinomas. They represent a degenerating process of the papillary stalks and are probably associated with a better prognosis.[1] Psammoma bodies are useful diagnostic clues in abdominal tumors of questionable origin, suggesting an ovarian primary origin (Fig. 6-13).

A small number of serous papillary carcinomas arise in adenofibromas, which are solid, firm tumors with abundant benign fibroconnective tissue (Fig. 6-14). An uncommon associated finding is squamous differentiation.[2]

## SEROUS PAPILLARY PERITONEAL CARCINOMA

Papillary serous carcinomas of the peritoneum are probably more common than generally thought. Some recent clinical reports[3,4] and immunohistochemical studies[5,6] have identified them as a subgroup of ovarian serous carcinomas in which the ovaries are either minimally or not at all involved.[7] The bulk of these tumors are found in the peritoneal cavity with massive involvement of the omentum, cul-de-sac, serosal surface of the uterus, bowel, urinary bladder, etc. Histologically, these tumors display papillary structures indentical to

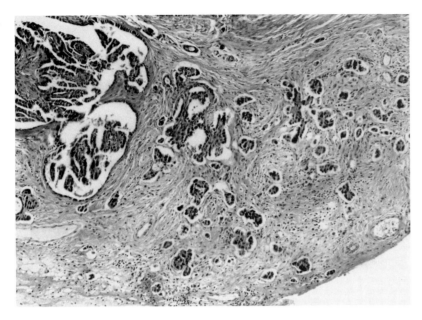

**Fig. 6-2** Same patient as in Fig. 6-1, opposite ovary. There is widespread dissemination of tumor in lymphatic channels. H&E, ×100.

those seen in the ovarian tumors, with an abundance of psammoma bodies.[5] Despite their origin in the peritoneal mesothelium, they are different from the mesotheliomas both clinically and microscopically:[6] they respond to chemotherapy in a similar fashion as the ovarian papillary carcinomas, and their antigenic expression is similar to that of müllerian epithelium rather than to that of the peritoneal mesothelium with which they share only some antigens.[5] These tumors arise from the mesothelium but have an epithelial phenotype.[8]

Grossly, the tumor masses located in the peritoneal cavity are whitish, firm, and sometime gritty because of the multiple calcifications (Plates 6-4 and 6-5). The ovaries may or may not be involved: the tumor can be focally present on the ovarian surface or sometime invade the ovarian cortex; grossly visible cystic tumor is usually absent. It has been arbitrarily established that the greatest diameter of the ovarian tumors is less than 4 cm.[3]

Microscopically, the papillary carcinomas are identical to the "classic" serous papillary ovarian tumors; psammoma bodies are abundant and represent a constant feature in the peritoneal tumors (Figs. 6-15 to 6-20).

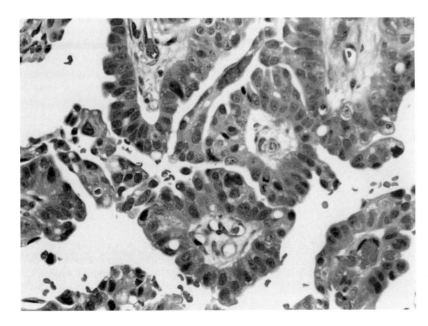

**Fig. 6-3** Grade 1 serous papillary carcinoma. Fibrovascular stalks are covered by neoplastic epithelial cells randomly arranged on several layers, displaying large pleomorphic nuclei and mitotic activity. H&E, ×400.

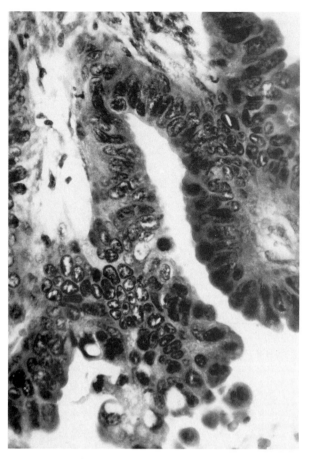

**Fig. 6-4** Grade 2 serous papillary carcinoma, showing malignant epithelial cells with high nuclear/cytoplasmic ratio, prominent and coarse chromatin network, intranuclear clearing, and mitoses. H&E, ×500.

## MUCINOUS CYSTADENOCARCINOMA

Mucinous adenocarcinomas are the third most frequent malignant ovarian tumors and represent about 8 to 10% of all primary ovarian malignancies.[9,10] The peak incidence of these tumors occurs between 40 and 60 years.

### GROSS PATHOLOGY

Mucinous adenocarcinomas are multilocular cystic tumors that may expand to very large dimensions (up to 50 cm in diameter). They are unilateral more often than the serous tumors, but bilateral more often than their benign counterparts, the mucinous cystadenomas. According to various series, their bilaterality ranges from 5 to 40%.[10] Their external surface is usually smooth, with round, bulging cysts, and the cut section exhibits a large number of cystic cavities of various sizes, filled with a jellylike grayish mucinous material. Solid areas are also present and represent the more diagnostically relevant areas to be sampled for histologic examination (Plate 6-6).

### MICROSCOPIC APPEARANCE

The basic pattern is that of glandular structures lined by tall, mucin–secreting epithelial cells, showing a back-to-back arrangement with little or no stroma between them. The individual cells display various degrees of

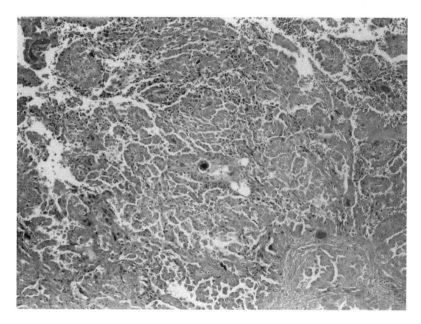

**Fig. 6-5** Ovarian moderately differentiated (grade 2) serous papillary carcinoma. Papillary structures show less connective tissue in stalks and more epithelial components. Note psammoma body in the center. H&E, ×40.

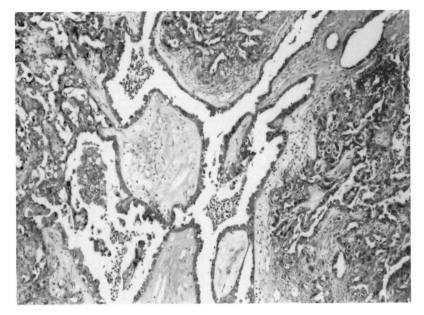

**Fig. 6-6** Grade 2 serous papillary carcinoma, showing coarse fibrovascular stalks and more solid epithelial elements. H&E, ×100.

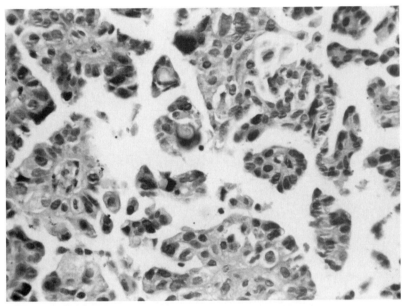

**Fig. 6-7** Grade 2 serous papillary carcinoma, showing papillary structures with little fibrovascular tissue. Epithelial cells display more nuclear pleomorphism than in the grade 1 tumors. A psammoma body is noted (upper center). H&E, ×200.

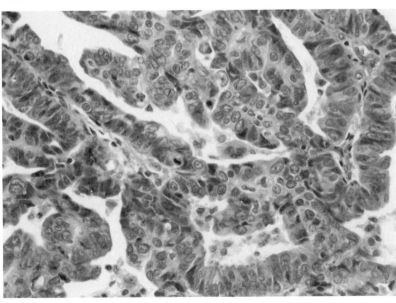

**Fig. 6-8** Grade 2 serous papillary carcinoma, showing papillary structures coalescing to form irregular nonglandular cavities. H&E, ×400.

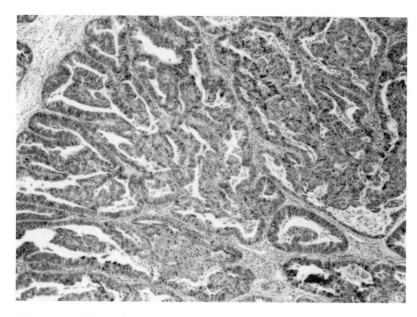

**Fig. 6-9** Grade 2 serous papillary carcinoma with papillary and glandular elements, reminiscent of endometrioid tumors. H&E, ×100.

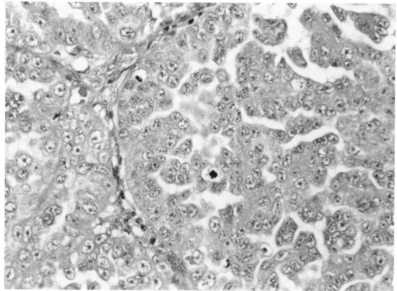

**Fig. 6-10** Poorly differentiated (grade 3) serous papillary carcinoma, a solid epithelial tumor with papillary features and scanty fibroconnective tissue. Tumor cells are poorly differentiated, with large nuclei containing prominent nucleoli and chromatin aggregates. H&E, ×400.

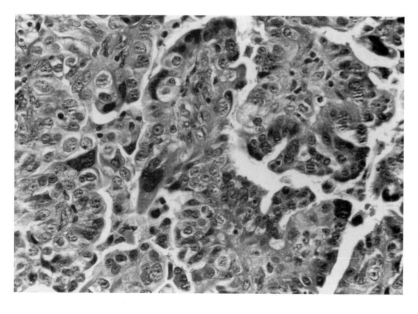

**Fig. 6-11** Grade 3 serous papillary carcinoma. Tumor cells are markedly pleomorphic displaying a wide variation in size, shape, and staining. Bizarre hyperchromatic nuclei are noted. H&E, ×400.

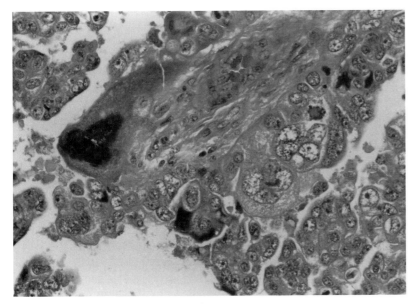

**Fig. 6-12** Grade 3 serous papillary carcinoma, showing bizarre multinucleated giant tumor cells along with severely pleomorphic cells exhibiting marked nuclear clearing and prominent nucleoli. H&E, ×1000.

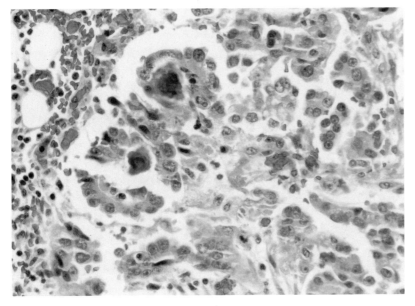

**Fig. 6-13** Tumor tissue from pelvis. Psammoma bodies in poorly differentiated carcinoma, suggestive of primary origin in ovary. H&E, ×400.

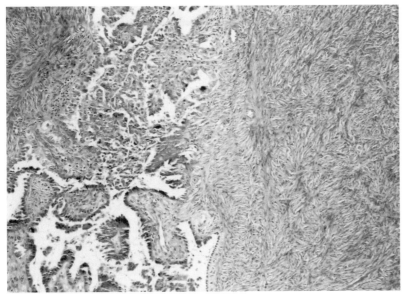

**Fig. 6-14** Ovarian serous papillary carcinoma arising in cystadenofibroma. Note benign lining merging with tumor (bottom, center). H&E, ×100.

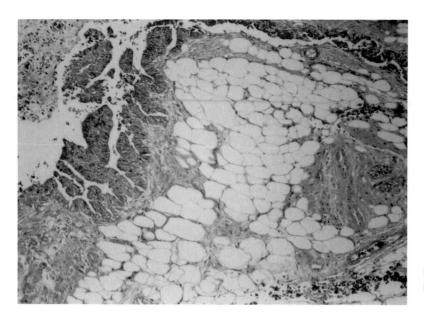

**Fig. 6-15** Extensive involvement of omentum by serous papillary carcinoma of peritoneum. H&E, ×100.

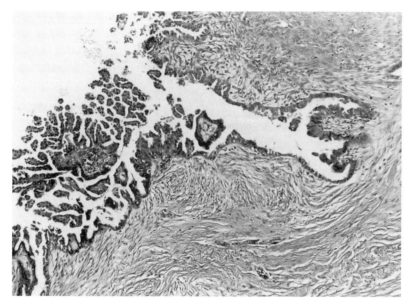

**Fig. 6-16** Serous papillary carcinoma of peritoneum involving pelvic wall. H&E, ×100.

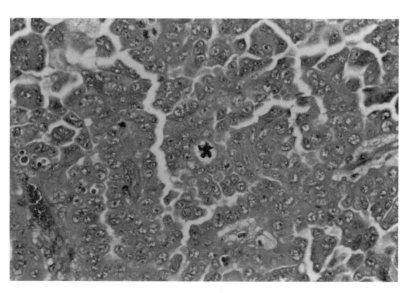

**Fig. 6-17** Grade 3 serous papillary carcinoma of peritoneum from bladder wall. Note marked nuclear pleomorphism and atypical mitosis (center). H&E, ×400.

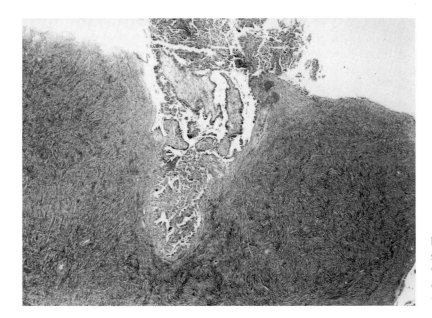

**Fig. 6-18** Same case as in Fig. 6-17, showing serous papillary carcinoma of peritoneum involving one grossly normal looking ovary focally, on the surface, with minimal cortical invasion. H&E, ×40.

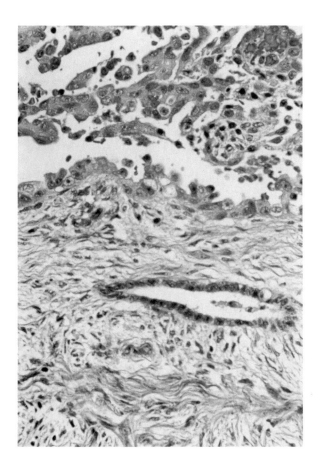

**Fig. 6-19** Serous papillary carcinoma of peritoneum, showing conglomerate of psammoma bodies (right upper corner) and benign epithelium in ovarian stroma. H&E, ×400.

anaplastic changes consisting of piling up, nuclear pleomorphism, loss of polarity, loss of cytoplasmic mucin content, and mitotic activity. The tumors are well differentiated (grade 1) when the glandular structures predominate; the epithelial lining is relatively regular with cytoplasmic apical mucin secretion (Figs. 6-21 and 6-22); moderately differentiated (grade 2) when solid areas of irregular tufts and sheets of epithelial cells with reduced mucin secretion are present (Figs. 6-23 to 6-25), and poorly differentiated (grade 3) when most of the tumor is solid with few glandular structures and minimal amounts of mucin are visible (Fig. 6-26); the grade 3 tumor cells are mostly arranged in nests and scattered clusters of cells, some with a "signet ring" appearance, not unlike adenocarcinomas of gastrointestinal origin. The mucinous cystadenocarcinomas are more often well differentiated and confined to the ovary than the serous papillary carcinomas.[9] Mixed epithelial serous and mucinous tumors are not uncommon (Fig. 6-27).

## PSEUDOMYXOMA PERITONEI

Pseudomyxoma peritonei is an accumulation of mucin pools in the peritoneal cavity that may occur with appendiceal and/or ovarian mucinous tumors. Histologically, single rows or incomplete glands lined by mucin-secreting epithelium are present (Fig. 6-28); they may be difficult to find because of the massive amount of mucinous material.

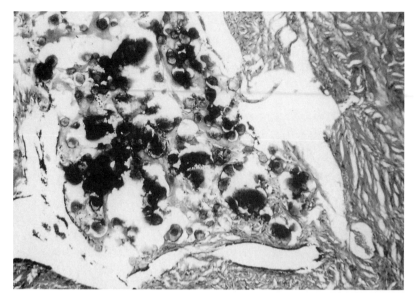

**Fig. 6-20** Serous papillary carcinoma of peritoneum, second look after chemotherapy. Pelvic wall biopsy shows abundant psammoma bodies. H&E, ×400.

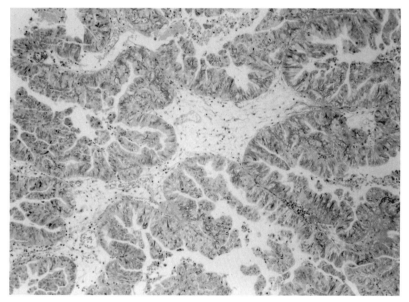

**Fig. 6-21** Ovarian mucinous cystadenocarcinoma, moderately differentiated (grade 2). Malignant glandular tumor diffusely infiltrates the ovary. H&E, ×100.

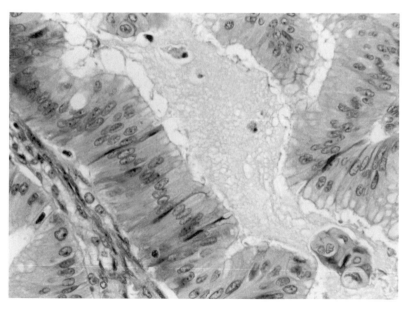

**Fig. 6-22** Grade 1 mucinous adenocarcinoma. Glands are lined by one or more rows of parallel epithelial cells showing abundant mucin secretion. Nuclei are relatively regular. H&E, ×400.

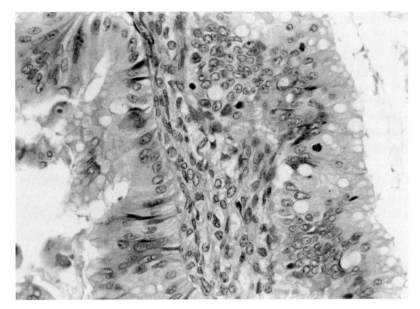

**Fig. 6-23** Ovarian mucinous adenocarcinoma grade 1. Malignant glands lined by relatively regular tall columnar epithelium with apical vacuoles containing mucin secretion. Lumen is filled by mucus. H&E, ×400.

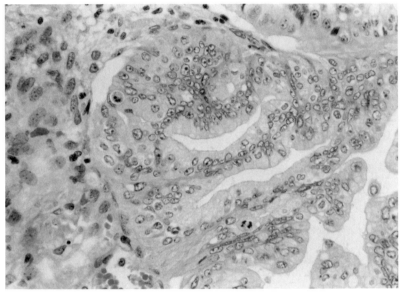

**Fig. 6-24** Grade 2 mucinous adenocarcinoma, showing partly solid, partly glandular tumor exhibiting loss of polarity of the epithelium, irregular epithelial tufts, and diminished mucin secretion. Mitoses are common. Note "clean" glandular lumen. H&E, ×250.

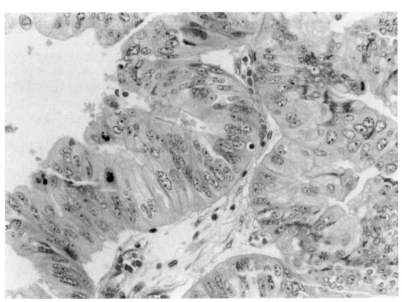

**Fig. 6-25** Grade 2 mucinous adenocarcinoma, showing piling up of epithelial cells, marked nuclear pleomorphism with prominent nucleoli, and coarse chromatin pattern, mitotic activity. H&E, ×250.

**97**

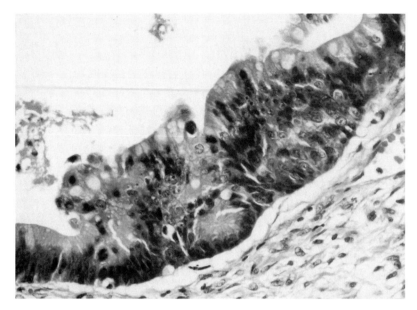

**Fig. 6-26** Grade 3 mucinous adenocarcinoma, showing piling up of glandular epithelium forming solid sheets of cells with high nuclear cytoplasmic ratio, marked nuclear atypia, and atypical mitoses. Mucin droplets are present only toward the lumen. H&E, ×400.

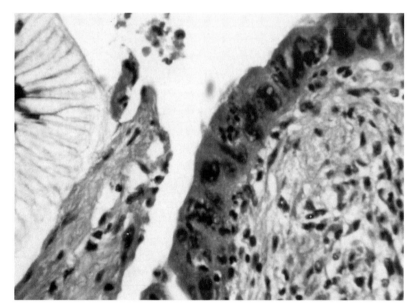

**Fig. 6-27** Mixed serous and mucinous cystadenocarcinoma; at left, mucin-secreting cells. H&E, ×500.

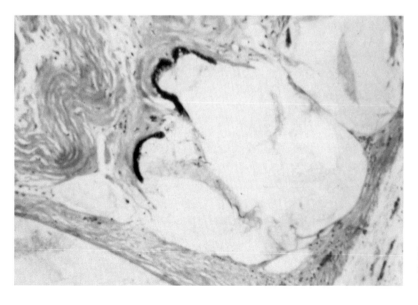

**Fig. 6-28** Pseudomyxoma peritonei, showing mucin pools and scanty single rows of epithelial cells. H&E, ×100.

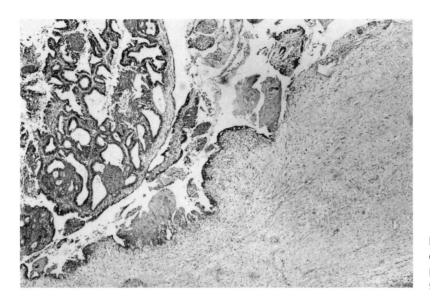

**Fig. 6-29** Endometrioid carcinoma arising in ovarian endometriosis. Squamoid metaplasia is present in both the tumor and the endometriosis. H&E, ×100.

## ENDOMETRIOID TUMORS

Endometrioid tumors are histologically identical to endometrial primary tumors and possibly arise in ovarian endometriosis. In some cases, their origin from benign endometriosis can be traced, with transition areas showing endometrial hyperplasia of various degrees of severity, analogous to the uterine adenomatous hyperplasia.[11,12] In most cases, however, the malignant tumor is ubiquitous with no histologically identifiable benign endometriosis. This tumor is the second most frequent malignant ovarian tumor, ranging between 16 and 31%.[10] The cancers arising in endometriotic cysts are usually seen in younger women and are often associated with primary endometrial neoplasms (adenomatous hyperplasia and/or well-differentiated adenocarcinoma).

## GROSS PATHOLOGY

Endometrioid carcinomas are slightly more often unilateral (about 55 to 60%). They are cystic and solid, sometime only solid, with friable brownish areas, and occasionally an adjacent "chocolate cyst" may be identified (Plate 6-7). Their external surface is smooth or granular, and their consistency is mostly soft. Sometime, a primary endometrial neoplasm is also present, usually noninvasive into the myometrium[13,14] (Plate 6-8). Criteria to rule out the possibility of an ovarian metastasis from the endometrial tumor include the finding of a multiple-nodule ovarian pattern and deep myometrial invasion.[15]

## MICROSCOPIC APPEARANCE

The histologic appearance is identical to that of the endometrial carcinomas: the basic pattern is that of a glandular malignant neoplasm (adenocarcinoma) in which the lining epithelium reproduces the müllerian epithelium with various degrees of differentiation. Squamoid elements are often present and may represent a diagnostic clue for the differential diagnosis from other abdominal tumors, especially from adenocarcinomas originating in the gastrointestinal tract (Fig. 6-29). Pure squamous cell carcinomas of the ovary are extremely uncommon. With rare exceptions,[16] they are presumed to arise in mature teratomas undergoing malignant transformation. Endometrioid carcinoma are some of the more often misdiagnosed ovarian tumors.

The endometrioid adenocarcinomas are lined by tall, pseudostratified epithelial cells displaying positive diastase-resistant PAS and mucicarmine stain at their apical border and elongated nuclei. They are well differentiated (grade 1) when the glandular pattern predominates (Figs. 6-30 and 6-31), moderately differentiated (grade 2) when solid tumor is present in about half of the representative sections (Fig. 6-32), and poorly differentiated (grade 3) when glandular structures are scant in a mostly solid tumoral mass (Fig. 6-33). The absence of glandular structures in the squamoid features should not be mistaken for solid tumor: bland-looking spindly or polygonal cells with intercellular bridges, low nuclear atypia, and low mitotic activity, similar to the "morules" described in adenomatous hyperplasia (Fig. 6-31) or well-differentiated endometrioid adenocarcinoma of the endometrium, may be associated with well-differentiated

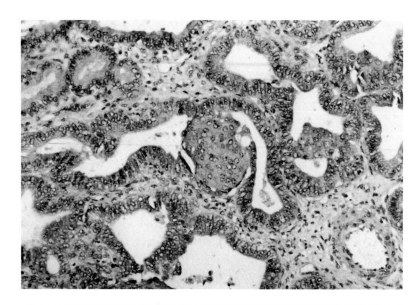

**Fig. 6-30** Well-differentiated endometrioid (grade 1) adenocarcinoma with squamoid "morule" (center). Tumor is similar to uterine adenocarcinoma. H&E, ×250.

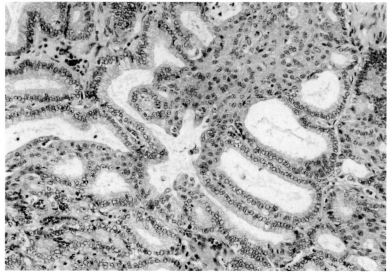

**Fig. 6-31** Well-differentiated (grade 1) endometrioid adenocarcinoma. Solid nest is composed of squamoid cells. H&E, ×200.

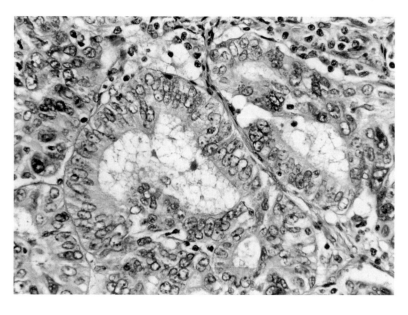

**Fig. 6-32** Moderately differentiated (grade 2) endometrioid carcinoma. Glandular epithelium is piled up; nuclei are pleomorphic with prominent nucleoli and coarse chromatin pattern. Note solid clusters of tumor cells. H&E, ×400.

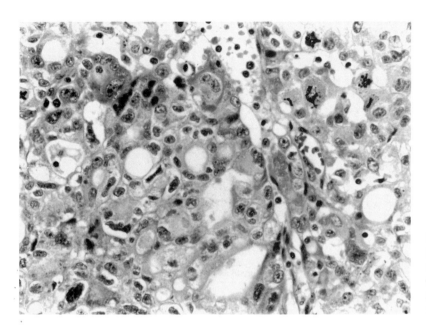

**Fig. 6-33** Poorly differentiated (grade 3) endometrioid adenocarcinoma, showing mostly solid tumor with some glandular structures. Cells are very pleomorphic and display highly atypical mitoses (right upper corner). H&E, ×400.

adenocarcinoma, as opposed to the anaplastic tumor cells, with bizarre, irregular nuclei and high mitotic activity seen in the solid tumor areas of poorly (Fig. 6-33) and moderately differentiated adenocarcinoma. Endometrioid carcinomas of the ovary should be differentiated from sex cord tumors and metastatic colonic carcinomas (Table 6-1). Immunohistochemistry is helpful in the differential diagnosis from sex cord and Sertoli cell tumors,[17] which also display less cellular atypia. Metastatic colonic carcinomas are characterized by intraglandular necrotic cellular debris and by marked cellular atypia seem with relative high glandular differentiation (Figs. 6-34 and 6-35) and are almost always bilateral. Mucinous metaplasia may occur in endometrioid carcinomas, as it does in endometrial adenocarcinoma.

## CLEAR CELL CARCINOMAS

The "pure" clear cell carcinomas are uncommon, representing 2 to 3% of all ovarian epithelial malignancies.[18] More often, they are associated with other histologic entities, especially with endometrioid carcinomas.[19] The mean age of the patients is the midfifties, and fewer than half of the tumors are bilateral.[10] *Grossly,* these are partly solid and partly cystic tumors, usually soft and friable, with necrotic areas. There are no particular gross characteristics for clear cell carcinomas. The origin of these tumors, once thought to be mesonephromas because of similarities to renal tumors, is in the müllerian-derived ovarian epithelium[9] and occasionally

**Table 6-1** Differential Diagnosis of Endometrioid Carcinoma

|  | *Endometrioid Carcinoma* | *Sex Cord Tumor* | *Metastatic Colonic Adenocarcinoma* |
| --- | --- | --- | --- |
| Bilateral tumors | Occasional | Rare | Frequent |
| Glandular structures | Present | Rare | Present |
| Mucin secretion | Scanty | Absent | Often present |
| Squamous elements | Present | Absent | Absent |
| Mucin at apical border | Present | Absent | Present |
| Necrotic material in lumen ("dirty glands") | Scant | Absent | Abundant |
| Goblet or signet ring cells | Absent | Absent | Occasional |
| Stratification | Few layers | Paired layers | Many layers |
| Epithelial membrane antigen | Positive | Negative | Positive |

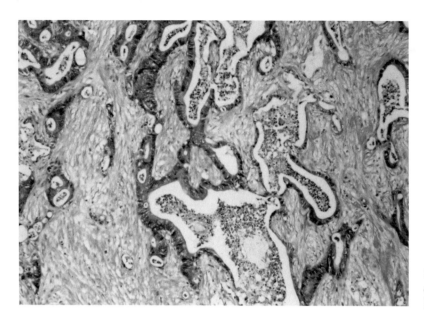

**Fig. 6-34** Metastatic colonic carcinoma to ovary. Glandular lumen contains necrotic debris. H&E, ×200.

in endometriosis, which is more commonly associated with this type of ovarian cancer.[18,20]

## MICROSCOPIC APPEARANCE

Glands, tubules, cystic spaces, and solid nests of malignant cells exhibiting an optically clear cytoplasm are characteristic (Fig. 6-36). The nuclei are pleomorphic and hyperchromatic and often protrude toward the lumen of glandular spaces forming papillary structures or hobnail patterns (Figs. 6-37 and 6-38). The clearing of the cytoplasm is due to glycogen accumulation, for

which special stains are positive, while other cells may display an eosinophilic granular cytoplasm. A rare variant is clear cell carcinoma in cystadenofibromas; this form is considered to be of borderline malignancy and has a better prognosis.[21]

## MALIGNANT MIXED MESODERMAL TUMORS

Malignant mixed mesodermal tumors (MMMTs) are composed of a mixture of malignant epithelial and ma-

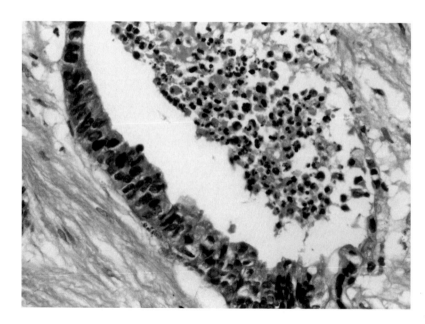

**Fig. 6-35** Metastatic colonic carcinoma to ovary. Glandular epithelium is markedly atypical; lumen contains necrotic debris and polymorphonuclear exudate. H&E, ×250.

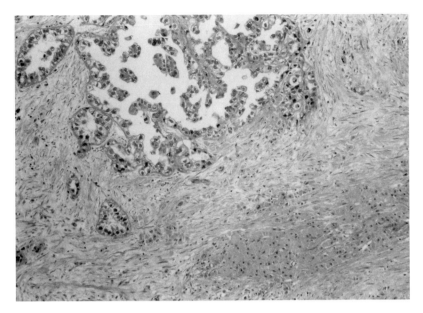

**Fig. 6-36** Ovarian clear cell carcinoma, showing glandular and papillary structures lined by tumor cells with clear cytoplasm. H&E, ×100.

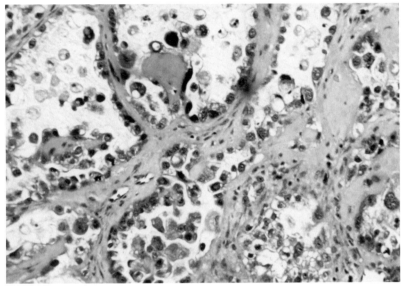

**Fig. 6-37** Clear cell carcinoma with hobnail cells, showing plump, irregular nuclei protruding toward the lumen. H&E, ×400.

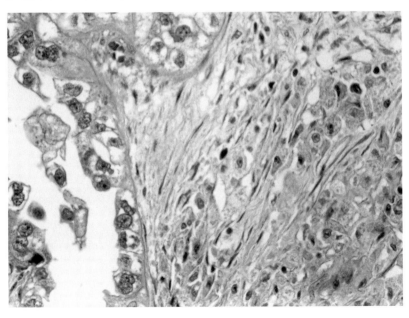

**Fig. 6-38** Clear cell carcinoma next to hemosiderin-laden macrophages, possibly from preceding endometriosis. H&E, ×400.

lignant mesenchymal cells. Also named mixed müllerian tumors, their designation as mixed mesodermal tumors is justified by the fact that they originate from the primitive mesodermal tissue from which both müllerian epithelium and stroma arise. More often encountered in the uterus, they are quite rare in the ovary, arising from the primitive coelomic epithelium and the adjacent ovarian stroma. Extensive sampling of serous papillary carcinoma occasionally discloses areas of mesenchymal malignancy.[22] Only rarely can their origin be traced from endometriosis, with malignant transformation of both the müllerian epithelium and stroma.[23] Most commonly, however, these tumors arise in elderly patients with no associated endometriosis and indicate a poor prognosis, with a more unfavorable outcome than that of patients with carcinomas of the same stage in both uterus and ovaries.[24-26] They are different from teratomas containing a mixture of malignant tissues: they occur in older patients and usually do not have organoid neuroectodermal tisues.[27]

Grossly, these tumors are large with necrotic and hemorrhagic areas and are mostly unilateral with cystic and solid areas. Their spread is similar to that of the malignant serous carcinomas, involving most commonly the peritoneum and occasionally abdominal organs (Plate 6-9).

### MICROSCOPIC APPEARANCE

Malignant epithelial and mesenchymal elements appear to be mixed and blend into each other. The epithelial structures are serous, papillary, glandular, or mucinous, occasionally with squamoid elements. If homologous, the mesenchymal malignant tissue is composed only of stromal elements, which can display a wide variety of bizarre and giant multinucleated cells (Figs. 6-39 to 6-41); if heterologous, malignant skeletal muscle (Fig. 6-42), cartilage, bone (Plate 6-10), or adipose tissues that are not normally seen in the uterus or ovary are noted. A diagnostic clue is the myxoid matrix (ground substance) (Fig. 6-43) in which the malignant mesenchymal elements are seen, occasionally with chondroid elements adjacent to tightly packed epithelial malignant cells. Immunohistochemical studies of intermediate filaments in these tumor cells identify mesenchymal and epithelial elements (Plates 6-11 to 6-13) as well as coexpression of both in anaplastic tumor cells.[26]

## ENDOMETRIOID STROMAL SARCOMAS

Endometrioid stromal sarcomas are very rare tumors and are high- or low-grade sarcomas, similar to those seen in the uterus. Low-grade stromal sarcomas are slightly more common. They may arise in endometriosis, are often widespread in the abdominal cavity, and occur in the fifth to sixth decade. Grossly, there may be multiple fleshy nodules involving ovaries and abdominal organs, with marked necrosis in the high-grade lesions. Histologically, the lesions are identical to those seen in uterine tumors. In the low-grade tumors, the cells show normal to oval nuclei, scant cytoplasm, and

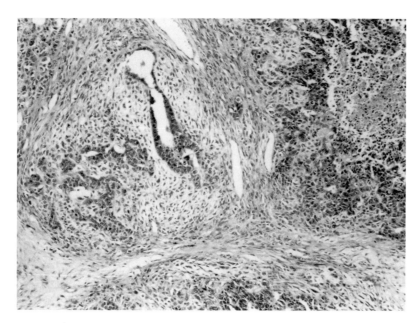

**Fig. 6-39** MMMT of ovary, composed of malignant epithelium with glandular differentiation and malignant mesenchymal tissue. H&E, ×100.

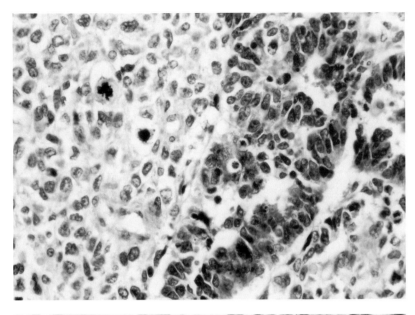

**Fig. 6-40** Homologous MMMT, showing malignant epithelium (right) and malignant stroma (left). H&E, ×400.

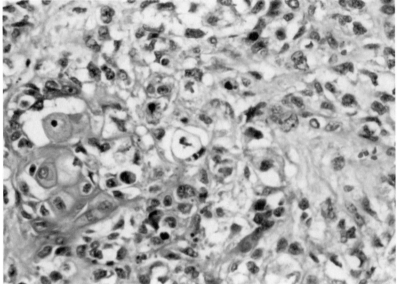

**Fig. 6-41** MMMT with squamous keratinizing elements (left). H&E, ×400.

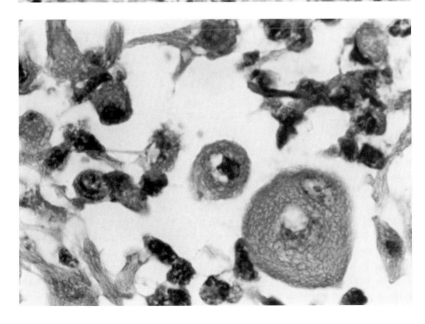

**Fig. 6-42** MMMT large rhabdomyoblasts with cytoplasmic cross striations. H&E, ×1000.

**105**

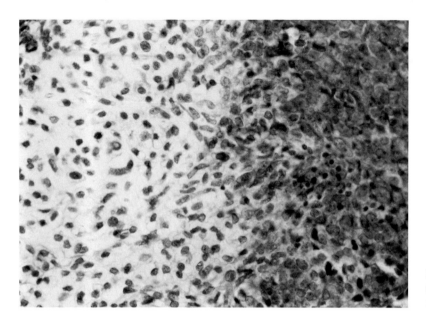

**Fig. 6-43** MMMT with minimal epithelial elements and myxoid chondroid stroma. H&E, ×400.

uncommon mitoses, along with marked vascularity (Fig. 6-44). In the high-grade tumors, nuclear atypia and mitotic activity are marked.[28,29]

## ADENOSARCOMAS

Adenosarcomas are very rare tumors in which in addition to the malignant stroma, benign epithelial elements are also present. They are unilateral and resemble histologically the uterine adenocarcinomas.

## MALIGNANT BRENNER TUMORS

Malignant Brenner tumors are very uncommon.[30,31] Grossly, they are mostly unilateral and are variable in size and consistency with solid and cystic areas. They are considered to be epithelial in origin.[32] Microscopically, these tumors are seen in continuity with benign or proliferating Brenner tumors (Fig. 6-45) and consist of infiltrating sheets of transitional, urothelial-type,[33] squamoid or anaplastic carcinoma, with occasional glandular structures. Mucinous adenocarcinoma may be associated. Their histologic and immunohistochemical

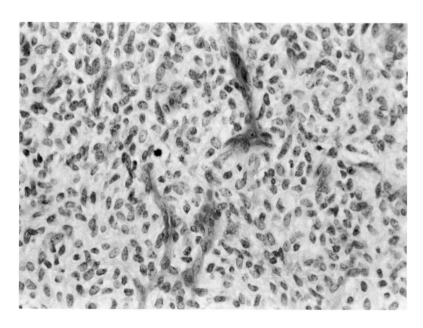

**Fig. 6-44** Ovarian low-grade stromal sarcoma with marked vascularity composed of relatively regular spindle-shaped cells and with few mitoses. H&E, ×400.

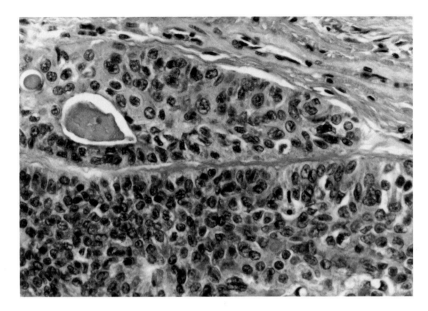

**Fig. 6-45** Malignant Brenner tumor with urothelial-type nests displaying some "coffee-bean nuclei." H&E, ×400.

characteristics have many common features with those of urinary bladder tumors.

## SMALL CELL CARCINOMA

Small cell carcinoma is an uncommon and very malignant ovarian cancer, seen in young women (under 40 years), often associated with hypercalcemia.[34,35] Grossly, most tumors are unilateral, fleshy, white-tan,

and solid with necrotic and hemorrhagic areas (Plate 6-14). Microscopically, they are composed of relatively uniform sheets and cords of small to intermediate cells, with scanty cytoplasm and hyperchromatic nuclei that have single nucleoli and display numerous mitoses (Figs. 6-46 and 6-47). Folliclelike structures are seen occasionally, simulating granulosa cell tumors. The epithelial nature of these tumors is supported by the positive stain for keratin and by electron microscopy,[35] although the resemblance of the tumor to a similar testicular tumor admixed with seminoma and teratoma raised the possibility of a germ cell origin.[36]

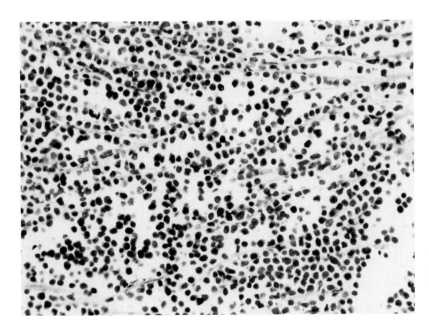

**Fig. 6-46** Small cell carcinoma showing sheets of relatively uniform tumor cells separated by thin collagen fibers. Patient was 32 years old, had no hypercalcemia, and survived only 8 months despite chemotherapy. H&E, ×250.

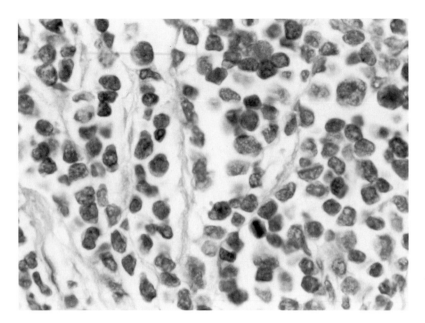

**Fig. 6-47** Same case as in Fig. 6-46, showing small to intermediate-sized tumor cells with scanty cytoplasm and hyperchromatic nuclei. H&E, ×400.

## UNDIFFERENTIATED AND UNCLASSIFIED CARCINOMAS

Undifferentiated and unclassified carcinomas are solid tumor masses showing necrosis and hemorrhage that microscopically display wide variations of cell size and shape. They are carcinomas because of their positive staining for epithelial cell markers (cytokeratin, Epithelial Membrane Antigen (EMA)) (Fig. 6-48). They may display some clear cell, glandular, squamoid, or urothelial features but do not qualify to be classified as such.[10,37,38]

One very uncommon variant is the hepatoid carcinoma,[39] which is not found in the context of a germ cell tumor with yolk sac differentiation but with other epithelial neoplasms such as endometrioid carcinoma (Figs. 6-49 and 6-50).

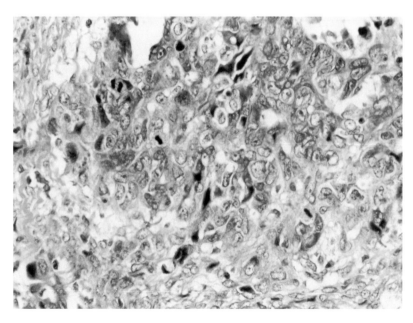

**Fig. 6-48** Undifferentiated carcinoma with no particular tissue pattern, showing anaplastic tumor cells staining positive for low-molecular-weight keratin and Epithelial Membrane Antigen. H&E, ×400.

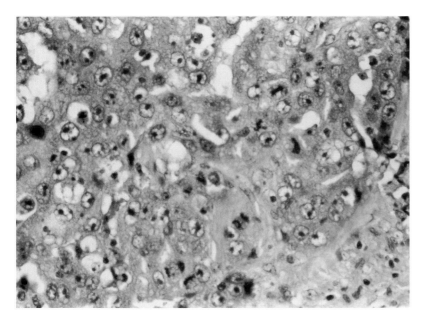

**Fig. 6-49** Ovarian poorly differentiated adenocarcinoma with hepatoid differentiation, staining positive for α-fetoprotein. Patient was 38 years old and survived 3 months. H&E, ×400.

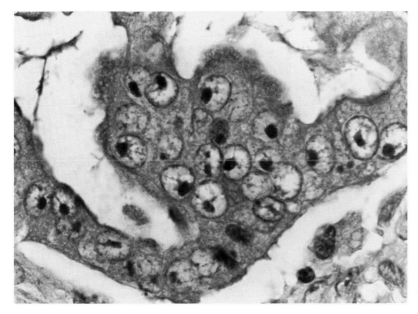

**Fig. 6-50** Same case as in Fig. 6-49. Opposite ovary with endometriotic cyst lined by atypical cells reminiscent of those of the tumor. H&E, ×1000.

## PLATES

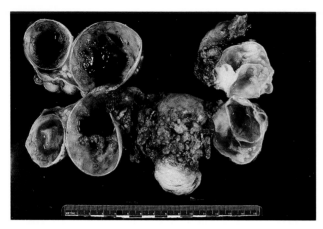

**Plate 6-1** Bilateral ovarian serous papillary cystadenocarcinoma. Tumor is also present on the external surface of the uterus.

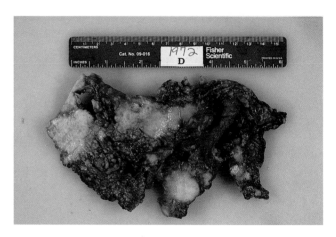

**Plate 6-4A** Serous papillary carcinoma of the peritoneum. Extensive omental involvement by tumor.

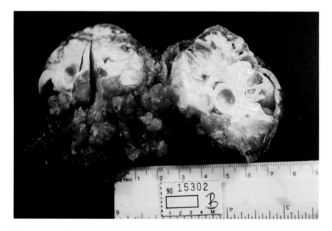

**Plate 6-2** Ovarian serous papillary carcinoma. Tumor is partly cystic, mostly solid with effacement of ovarian structures.

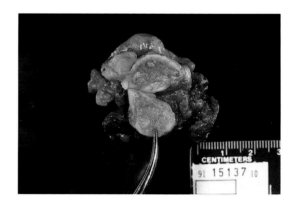

**Plate 6-4B** Minimally involved ovary, same case.

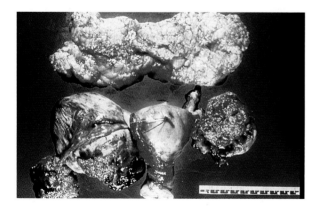

**Plate 6-3** Bilateral ovarian serous papillary carcinoma with extensive omental involvement (stage III).

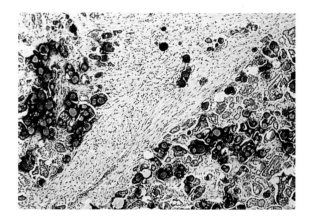

**Plate 6-5** Abundant psammoma bodies in serous papillary carcinoma of peritoneum. H&E, ×100.

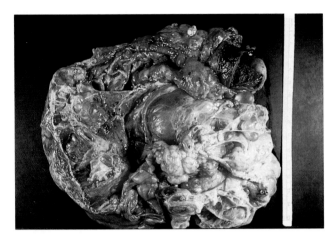

**Plate 6-6** Large ovarian mucinous cystadenocarcinoma. Malignant tumor is mostly seen in the solid areas.

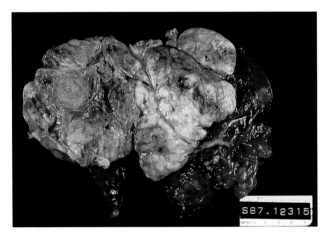

**Plate 6-9** MMMT metastatic to spleen.

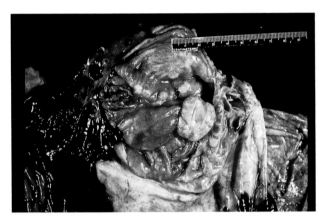

**Plate 6-7** Endometriosis of ovary ("chocolate cyst") and solid tumor (endometrioid adenocarcinoma).

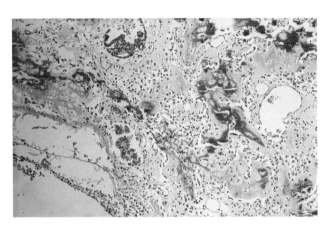

**Plate 6-10** MMMT, heterologous, showing bone tissue with malignant mesenchymal and epithelial components. H&E, ×100.

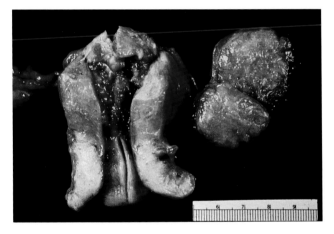

**Plate 6-8** Ovarian endometrioid adenocarcinoma and separate primary endometrial tumor.

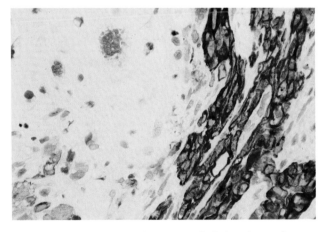

**Plate 6-11** MMMT, heterologous. Epithelial and rare chondroid tumor cells staining positive for cytokeratin. H&E, ×250.

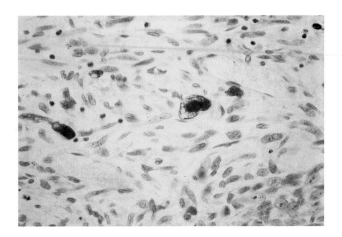

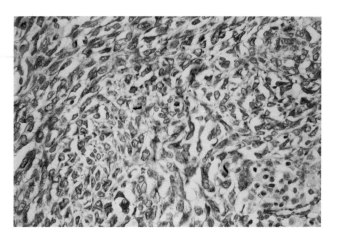

**Plate 6-12** Heterologous MMMT. Rhabdomyoblasts stain positive for myoglobin. × 400.

**Plate 6-13** Homologous MMMT showing diffuse positive staining for vimentin. × 250.

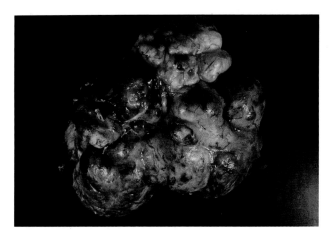

**Plate 6-14** Small cell carcinoma of ovary.

## REFERENCES

1. Aure JC, Hoeg K, Kalstad P. Psammoma bodies in serous carcinoma of the ovary: A prognostic study. *Am J Obstet Gynecol* 109:113–118, 1971.
2. Ulbright TM, Roth LM, Sutton GP. Papillary serous carcinoma of the ovary with squamous differentiation. *Int J Gynecol Pathol* 9:86–94, 1990.
3. Fromm GL, Gershenson DM, Silva EG. Papillary serous carcinoma of the peritoneum. *Obstet Gynecol* 75:89–95, 1990.
4. August CZ, Murad TM, Newton M. Multiple focal extra-ovarian serous carcinoma. *Int J Gynecol Pathol* 4:11–23, 1985.
5. Wick MR, Mills SE, Dehner LP, Bollinger DJ, Fechner RE. Serous papillary carcinomas arising from the peritoneum and ovaries. A clinico-pathologic and immunohistochemical comparison. *Int J Gynecol Pathol* 8:179–188, 1989.
6. Raju U, Fine G, Greenwald KA, Ohorodnik JM. Primary papillary serous neoplasm of the peritoneum: A clinicopathologic and ultrastructural study of eight cases. *Hum Pathol* 20:426–436, 1989.
7. Feuer GA, Shevchuk M, Calanog A. Normal sized ovary carcinoma syndrome. *Obstet Gynecol* 73:78–92, 1988.
8. Truong LD, Maccato ML, Awalt H. Serous surface carcinoma of the peritoneum: A clinico-pathologic study of 22 cases. *Hum Pathol* 21:99–110, 1990.
9. Scully RE. *Tumors of the Ovary and Maldeveloped Gonads.* Atlas of Tumor Pathology, second series, fascicle 16. Washington, DC, Armed Forces Institute of Pathology, pp 61–64, 1979.
10. Czernobilsky B. Common epithelial tumors of the ovary. In *Blaustein's Pathology of the Female Genital Tract.* 3d ed. New York Ed. Kurman Springer-Verlag, 1987, pp 453–504.
11. LaGrenade A, Silverberg SG. Ovarian tumors associated with atypical endometriosis. *Hum Pathol* 19:1080–1084, 1988.
12. Moll UM, Chumas JC, Chalas E. Ovarian carcinoma arising in atypical endometriosis. *Obstet Gynecol* 75:537–539, 1988.
13. Eisner RF, Nieberg RK, Berek JS. Synchronous primary neoplasms of the female reproductive tract. *Gynecol Oncol* 33:335–339, 1988.
14. Tidy J, Mason WP. Endometrioid carcinoma of the ovary: A retrospective study. *Br J Obstet Gynecol* 95:1165–1169, 1988.
15. Ulbright TM, Roth LM. Metastatic and independent cancers of the endometrium and ovary: A clinico-pathologic study of 34 cases. *Hum Pathol* 16:28–34, 1985.
16. Tetu B, Silva EG, Gershenson DM. Squamous cell carcinoma of the ovary. *Arch Pathol Lab Med* 111:864–866, 1987.
17. Aguirre P, Thor AD, Scully RE. Ovarian endometrioid carcinomas resembling sex cord–stromal tumors. An immunohistochemical study. *Int J Gynecol Pathol* 8:364–73, 1989.
18. Crozier MA, Copeland LJ, Silva EG. Clear cell carcinoma of the ovary: A study of 59 cases. *Gynecol Oncol* 35:199–203, 1989.
19. Brescia RJ, Dubin N, Demopoulos RI. Endometrioid and clear cell carcinoma of the ovary: Factors affecting survival. *Int J Gynecol Pathol* 8:132–138, 1989.
20. Jenison EL, Montag AG, Griffiths CT. Clear cell carcinoma of the ovary: A clinical analysis and comparison with serous carcinoma. *Gynecol Oncol* 32:65–71, 1989.
21. Bell DA, Scully RE. Benign and borderline clear cell adenofibroma of the ovary. *Cancer* 56:2922–2931, 1985.
22. Noorduyn LA, Herman CJ. The relation between mixed mesodermal tumors and adenocarcinomas of the ovary. An immunopathologic study. *Eur J Cancer Clin Oncol* 23:157–162, 1987.
23. Saunders P, Price AB. Mixed mesodermal tumor of the ovary arising in pelvic endometriosis. *Proc R Soc Med* 63:1050–1053, 1970.
24. Barwick KW, LiVolsi VA. Malignant mixed mesodermal tumors of the ovary: A clinico-pathologic assessment of 12 cases. *Am J Surg Pathol* 4:37–42, 1980.
25. Morrow CP, D'Ablaing G, Brady LW. A clinical and pathologic study of 30 cases of malignant mixed müllerian epithelial and mesenchymal tumors: A gynecologic oncology group study. *Gynecol Oncol* 18:278–292, 1984.
26. Deligdisch L, Plaxe S, Cohen CJ. Extrauterine pelvic malignant mixed mesodermal tumors: A study of 10 cases with immunohistochemistry. *Int J Gynecol Pathol* 7:361–372, 1988.
27. Calame JJ, Schaberg A. Solid teratomas and mixed müllerian tumors of the ovary: A clinical, histological and immunocytochemical comparative study. *Gynecol Oncol* 33:212–221, 1989.
28. Shakfeh SM, Woodruff JD. Primary ovarian sarcomas: Report of 46 cases and review of the literature. *Obstet Gynecol Surv* 42:331–349, 1987.
29. Silverberg SG, Fernandez FN. Endolymphatic stromal myosis of the ovary: A report of three cases and literature review. *Gynecol Oncol* 12:129–138, 1981.
30. Roth LM, Czernobilsky B. Ovarian Brenner tumors: II. Malignant. *Cancer* 56:592–601, 1985.
31. Miles PA, Norris JH. Proliferation and malignant Brenner tumors of the ovary. *Cancer* 30:174–186, 1972.
32. Trebeck CE, Friedlander ML, Russell P. Brenner tumors of the ovary: A study of the histology, immunohistochemistry and cellular DNA content in benign, borderline, and malignant ovarian tumors. *Pathology* 19:241–246, 1987.
33. Aguirre P, Scully RE, Wolfett J. Argyrophil cells in Brenner tumors: Histochemical and immunohistochemical analysis. *Int J Gynecol Pathol* 5:223–234, 1986.
34. Pruett KM, Gordon AN, Estrada R. Small carcinoma of the ovary: An aggressive epithelial cancer occurring in young patients. *Gynecol Oncol* 29:365–369, 1988.
35. Abeler V, Kjrstad KE, Nesland JM. Small cell carcinoma of the ovary: A report of six cases. *Int J Gynecol Pathol* 7:315–329, 1988.
36. Ulbright TM, Roth LM, Stehman FB. Poorly differentiated (small cell) carcinoma of the ovary in young women:

Evidence supporting a germ cell origin. *Hum Pathol* 18: 175–184, 1987.

37. Silva EG, Tornos C, Bailey MA. Undifferentiated carcinoma of the ovary. *Arch Pathol Lab Med* 15:377–381, 1991.

38. Russel P, Bannatyne P. *Surgical Pathology of the Ovaries.* Edinburgh, Churchill Livingstone, 1989, pp 294–295.

39. Ishikura H, Scully RE. Hepatoid carcinoma of the ovary. A newly described tumor. *Cancer* 60:2775–2784, 1987.

# 7

# Preinvasive Epithelial Ovarian and Peritoneal Malignancy

*Liane Deligdisch, M.D.*

Precursor lesions of cervical and endometrial uterine malignancies have been extensively studied and their histogenesis as well as risk factors (viral for the cervix, hormonal for the endometrium) have been widely documented. This has contributed to a dramatic decrease in morbidity and mortality due to uterine cancer. For ovarian cancer, on the other side, not only are the precursor lesions poorly understood, but the early invasive stages are rarely diagnosed.

Most ovarian malignant tumors are of epithelial origin. About 85% of patients present in stage III of their disease, with tumor spread to the pelvic and abdominal cavity. Usually, they become symptomatic when the neighboring organs are involved. The morbidity and mortality due to ovarian cancer is the highest of all female pelvic malignant tumors.

The early stages of ovarian carcinoma are rarely diagnosed, and preinvasive histologic lesions were described only recently.[1-3] Premalignant, noninvasive lesions have been studied in most epithelial neoplasms (larynx, colon, cervix, etc.) in the vicinity of overt invasive cancer. Identification of their histologic characteristics has been used for screening the population at risk. Because of the secluded location of the ovaries and their difficult accessibility, a screening based on cytologic and histologic patterns is still elusive. With the application of new surgical techniques, especially laparoscopy, the ovaries become more accessible and an extensive study of tissue samples may offer the necessary insight into

early dysplastic, preinvasive malignant and early invasive lesions.

Prophylactic oophorectomies done on identical twin sisters of women with ovarian carcinoma revealed microscopic changes of the ovarian surface epithelium consisting of stratification, loss of polarity, and nuclear pleomorphism, with prominent nucleoli and a coarse chromatin pattern (Figs. 7-1 and 7-2).[4] These histologic changes are consistent with dysplastic changes seen in other epithelial tissues, in which precursors of invasive cancer have been documented (uterine cervix, larynx, gallbladder, etc.).

The tissue directly adjacent to the overt tumor from cases of stage I ovarian carcinoma was screened for histologic features involving tissue architecture and nuclear characteristics consistent with dysplasia (Figs. 7-3 to 7-5). The changes in tissue architecture (stratification and loss of polarity) (Figs. 7-6 to 7-8) and in nuclear profiles (increased nuclear/cytoplasmic ratio, pleomorphism, hyperchromasia, and irregular chromatin distribution) (Figs. 7-9 and 7-10) were similar to those described in the ovarian epithelium from nontumoral ovaries removed by preventive oophorectomy in some high-risk patients (identical twin sisters of patients with ovarian carcinoma).

In order to enhance the accuracy of the diagnosis of these histologic changes, ovarian dysplastic changes were evaluated by computerized image analysis. Morphometric studies were performed in order to assess the

**115**

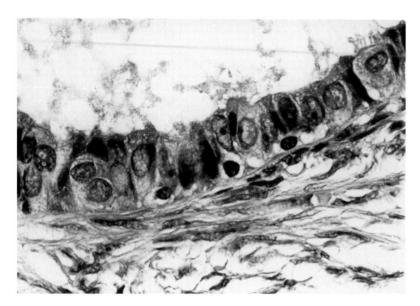

**Fig. 7-1** Dysplastic epithelium lining grossly normal looking ovary removed by prophylactic oophorectomy from an identical twin sister of a patient with ovarian carcinoma. Note nuclear pleomorphism and loss of polarity. H&E, ×1000.

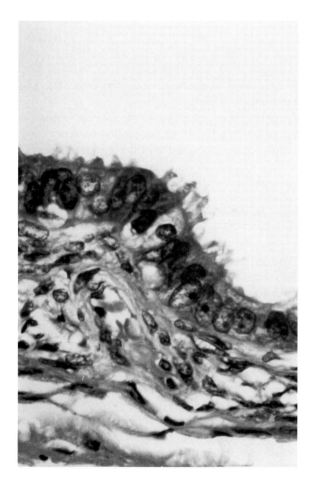

**Fig. 7-2** Dysplastic epithelium adjacent to ovarian carcinoma: note stratification, loss of polarity, nuclear pleomorphism with prominent nucleoli, and coarse chromatin pattern, quite similar to changes seen in Fig. 7-1. H&E, ×1000.

architectural and cytologic characteristics of the ovarian surface epithelium; computerized image analysis was particularly suitable because of the quantifiable criteria used to define ovarian dysplasia. This way, the subjective evaluation of histologic patterns was tested by an objective method that included a multivariate statistical analysis.

Morphometry was performed on tissue from normal ovaries, from ovarian carcinoma, and from ovarian lesions characterized as dysplastic by histologic criteria (Figs. 7-11 to 7-13). Two different interactive procedures were used, one for the architectural changes, measuring the degree of stratification and nuclear crowding (Fig. 7-14), the other measuring nuclear profiles (surface area, perimeter length, maximal chord, and circularity index) (Fig. 7-15). These procedures were performed on histologic slides projected on a video machine with a touch-sensitive screen.[1,3] Tracing basement membranes and measuring the shortest distance to the nuclear center of the epithelium above the basement membrane was followed by computation of number of nuclei per millimeter of basement membrane, thus evaluating the nuclear crowding. Mean values of nuclear crowding were found to be 159.4 per 1 mm of basement membrane in normal epithelium, 241 in dysplasia, and 400.2 in malignancy. Stratification measured by mean distances of nuclei from the basement membrane was 33 $\mu$m in normal epithelium, 78 $\mu$m in dysplastic epithelium, and 150 $\mu$m in malignancy.[1]

Tracing of the nuclear profiles evaluates the nuclear pleomorphism. Mean nuclear area was 22.7 $\mu m^2$ in normal, 44.9 $\mu m^2$ in dysplastic, and 70 $\mu m^2$ in malignant nuclei. Maximal chord length was 7.8, 12.88, and 16.10

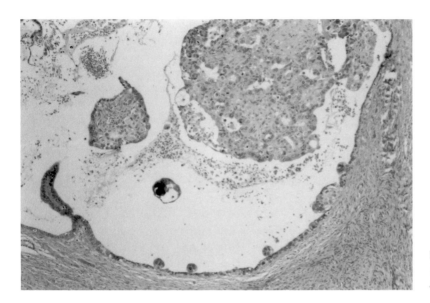

**Fig. 7-3** Stage I grade 1 ovarian serous papillary carcinoma. Dysplastic changes were found adjacent to the tumor. H&E, ×40.

μm, respectively. The class distribution subdividing nuclear area into 10 groups ("bins") showed the characteristic "malignant tail": the group including the largest nuclear area (above 90 μm) was high in cancer cells, low in dysplastic cells, and absent in normal cells. The multivariate statistical analysis included the above-described factors, their standard deviations, and a subdivision of the size distribution into 10 subgroups for both the architectural (measuring distances from nuclei to basement membrane) and the cytologic (measuring nuclear areas) features. The statistical analysis based on this large number of variables proved to be highly accurate, judging from the resulting "posterior probabilities."[1,3]

The morphometric studies achieved a clear-cut discrimination between the three diagnostic categories;

normal, dysplastic, and malignant ovarian epithelium. A database was created showing the consistency of the three diagnostic categories. On this basis, ovarian dysplasia, or ovarian intraepithelial neoplasia (OIN), becomes an acceptable histologic entity.

Ovarian dysplasia, or OIN,[2] can be defined as a lesion characterized histologically by crowding and piling up of epithelial cells, and loss of polarity; the nuclei have a statistically significant larger surface area, larger maximal chord, and larger perimeter length than normal ovarian surface epithelium.

The natural history of these lesions, as in dysplasias of other epithelial tissues, is unpredictable. Whether there will be a progression to overt malignancy, arrest, or regression depends on a number of yet poorly under-

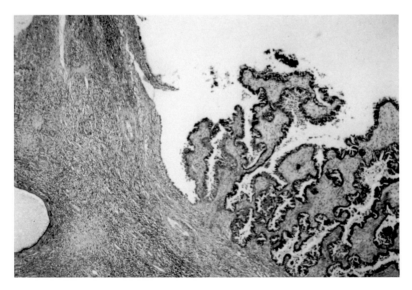

**Fig. 7-4** Stage I grade 1 ovarian serous papillary carcinoma. Screening for dysplastic changes was done in the epithelial lining adjacent to the tumor. H&E, ×100.

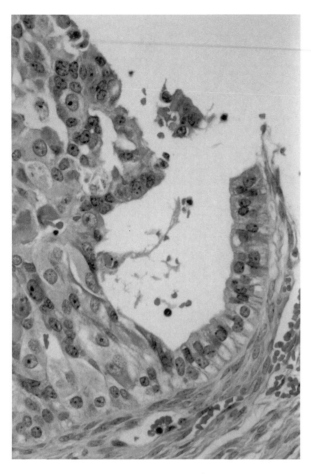

**Fig. 7-5** Dysplastic epithelium (right) adjacent to ovarian stage I grade 2 carcinoma (left). High magnification. H&E, ×400.

stood factors, mostly regarding the host's defense mechanism. Their identification, however, is the basis of any screening program. These changes are often encountered in epithelial inclusion cysts associated with overt carcinoma, frequently next to psammoma bodies. In ovaries with no overt cancer, these changes may represent a potential precancerous lesion and justify a closer follow-up of the patient. The morphologic features seem to be more significant, at the present time, than the rather insensitive and nonspecific tumor markers.[5,6]

Preinvasive (dysplastic or intraepithelial neoplastic) ovarian lesions have to be distinguished from "borderline" or LMP ovarian tumors that are also not invasive but represent a full-blown neoplastic process with a well-documented natural history. One common characteristic of both borderline and malignant ovarian lesions is their propensity for peritoneal spread. Because of the common embryologic heritage of the ovarian surface epithelium and coelomic mesothelium, a "field effect" of carcinogenic agents has been postulated.[7,8,9,10]

Borderline ovarian tumors are associated with peritoneal implants in about 15 to 20% of the cases. After bilateral oophorectomy and chemotherapy, patients with ovarian carcinoma develop recurrences on the peritoneum that are often difficult to distinguish from mesothelial hyperplasia. Is there a dysplasia of the peritoneal mesothelium that precedes the overt carcinoma? Or is the peritoneal cancer a metastatic secondary deposit of tumor?

Morphometric studies have compared mesothelial hyperplasia and ovarian dysplasia, in parallel with the comparative measurements performed in malignant

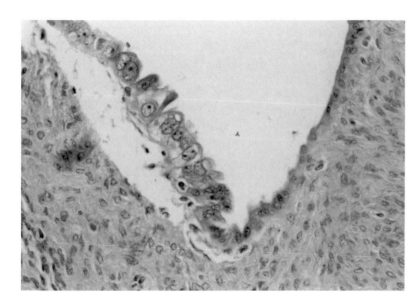

**Fig. 7-6** Dysplastic epithelium (left) adjacent to normal ovarian epithelium. Note stratification and loss of polarity. H&E, ×400.

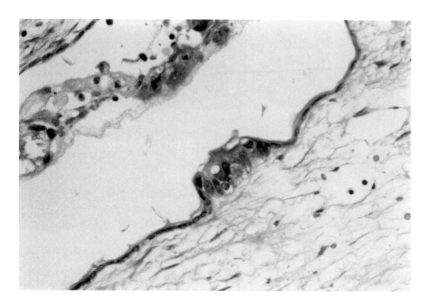

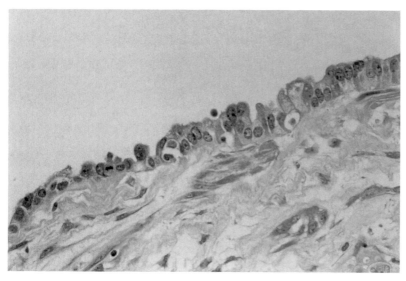

**Fig. 7-7** Cluster of dysplastic cells (center) and adjacent normal ovarian epithelium. H&E, ×400.

**Fig. 7-8** Ovarian intraepithelial neoplasia, displaying stratification, loss of polarity, and occasional mitosis. H&E, ×250.

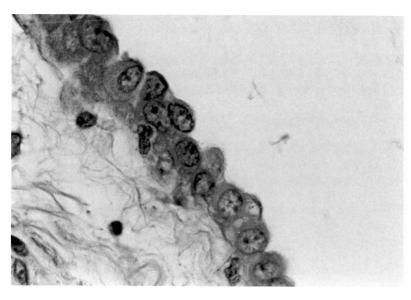

**Fig. 7-9** Nuclear profile changes in ovarian dysplasia, or ovarian intraepithelial neoplasia, included increased nuclear/cytoplasmic ratio, pleomorphism, and irregular chromatin distribution, seen in the vicinity of ovarian carcinoma. H&E, ×400.

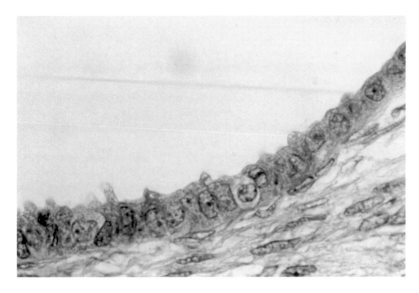

**Fig. 7-10** Nuclear profiles from a high-risk patient who underwent preventive oophorectomy. Note similarity to the features seen in Fig. 7-9. H&E, ×400.

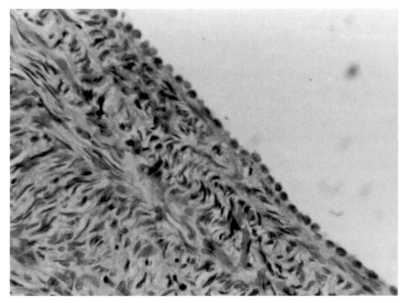

**Fig. 7-11** Normal ovarian surface epithelium, used for morphometry. H&E, ×40.

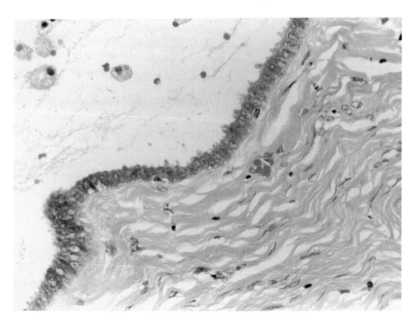

**Fig. 7-12** Dysplastic ovarian surface epithelium, used for morphometry. H&E, ×40.

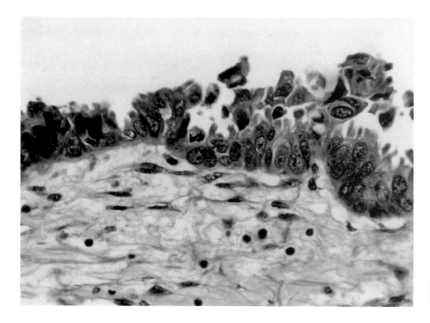

**Fig. 7-13** Malignant ovarian surface epithelium, used for morphometry. H&E, ×100.

(ovarian and peritoneal) and normal (ovarian and mesothelial) tissues.[11] Despite some similarities evident at the microscopic examination such as clustering, increased nuclear/cytoplasmic ratio, and nuclear hyperchromasia of the hyperplastic mesothelium, dysplastic changes can be identified on the basis of the marked difference in the size distribution of their nuclei. In mesothelial hyperplasia, most cells averaged 20 to 50 $\mu m^2$, while dysplastic cell nuclei were more pleomorphic, being distributed throughout all size groups, from 10 to 90 $\mu m^2$.

In analogy with cervical uterine lesions, a comparison could be drawn between squamous metaplasia and mesothelial hyperplasia on one side, and squamous dysplasia or Cervical Intraepithelial Neoplasia (CIN) and ovarian dysplasia (OIN) on the other side. While the benign hyperplastic and metaplastic changes show enlarged nuclei, crowding, and piling up, a certain uniformity in the size and shape of the cell nuclei is characteristic (Figs. 7-16 and 7-17). Dysplastic changes show a lack of uniformity that has been objectively confirmed

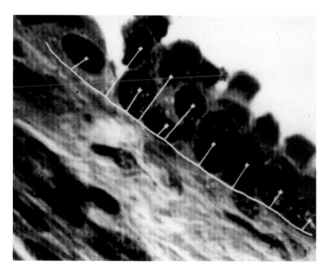

**Fig. 7-14** Interactive morphometric procedure used for determining architectural changes of dysplastic epithelium, measuring distance of nuclei from the basement membrane (stratification) and their number per unit of basement membrane (crowding).

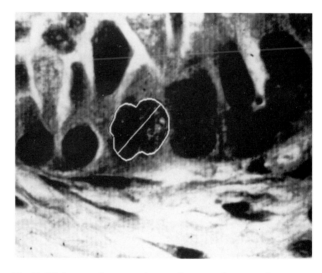

**Fig. 7-15** Interactive morphometric procedure used to measure nuclear profiles (perimeter length, area, and maximal chord).

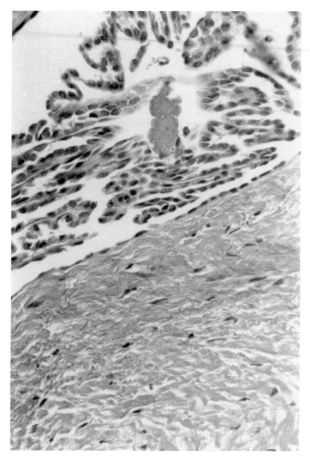

**Fig. 7-16** Benign hyperplasia of peritoneal mesothelium exhibiting crowding and piling up of cells. H&E, ×100.

by morphometry, based on the nuclear size distribution (Fig. 7-18). The discrimination between mesothelial hyperplasia and dysplasia can be helpful in identifying precursors of peritoneal carcinoma, which may arise from local mesothelium rather than representing a metastasis from the ovary.

In the peritoneal cavity, lesions designated as *endosalpingiosis, müllerian remnants* with or without atypia consisting of tubular structures lined by cuboidal to columnar epithelium (Fig. 7-19) are often the object of controversies and may represent a diagnostic dilemma, especially in patients receiving chemotherapy for ovarian cancer. Their epithelial or mesothelial lining is somewhat similar to that of the frequently seen epithelial "inclusions" of the ovary (Figs. 7-20 and 7-21). Various degrees of atypia are often present in their epithelial lining, but to what extent they may represent potential precursors of cancer is unknown (Figs. 7-22 to 7-24). In second-look operations for ovarian cancer, when the finding of residual or recurrent foci of cancer is of great significance for the management of the patient, the differential diagnosis between endosalpingiosis, mesothelial hyperplasia, carcinoma responding to chemotherapy, or dysplasia is not always an easy one. Morphometric analysis has proved helpful in creating objective discriminating criteria for this important differential diagnosis and for differentiating tumor cells responsive to chemotherapy from nonresponsive ones (Figs. 7-25 to 7-27).[12] Further improvements, such as the use of nuclear texture evaluating the chromatin pattern (Fig. 7-28) and nucleolar organizers[13] add accu-

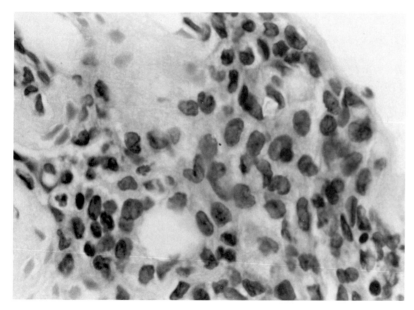

**Fig. 7-17** Benign hyperplasia of peritoneal mesothelium. Nuclear/cytoplasmic ratio is increased and the nuclei are uniformly enlarged. H&E, ×400.

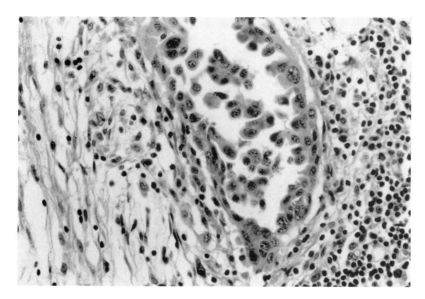

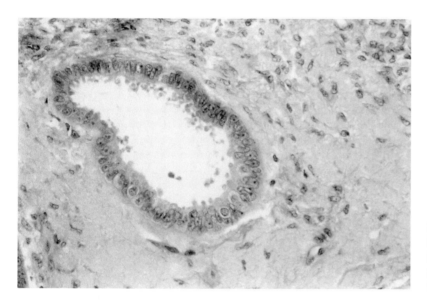

Fig. 7-18 Peritoneal mesothelial cell proliferation associated with ovarian serous papillary carcinoma. Computerized image analysis classified these cells as dysplastic. Note coarse chromatin pattern and irregular size distribution of the nuclei. H&E, ×100.

Fig. 7-19 "Endosalpingiosis." Tubular structure lined by cuboidal to columnar epithelium. Some cells are ciliated; others show pale cytoplasm, reminiscent of the fallopian tube epithelium. H&E, ×100.

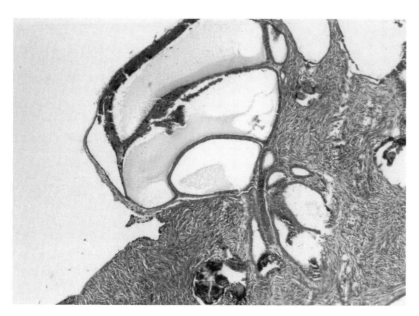

Fig. 7-20 Multiple ovarian epithelial inclusion cysts, with psammoma bodies in their vicinity. H&E, ×40.

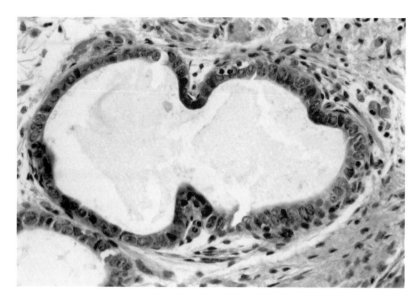

**Fig. 7-21** Ovarian epithelial inclusion cyst lined by cuboidal to columnar epithelium, similar to the extraovarian endosalpingiosis. H&E, ×100.

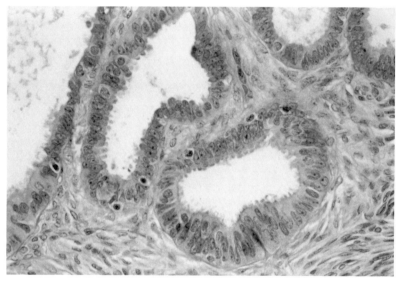

**Fig. 7-22** Ovarian epithelial inclusion cysts showing cell proliferation with mild atypia. H&E, ×100.

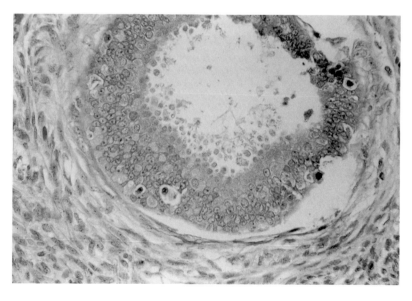

**Fig. 7-23** Ovarian epithelial inclusion cysts displaying stratification, some of it due to tangential cut section, and mitotic figures. H&E, ×100.

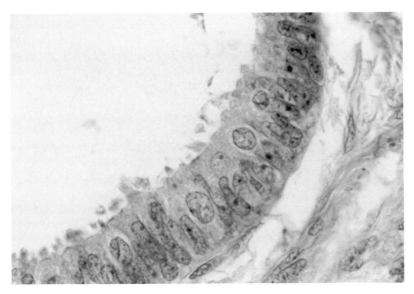

**Fig. 7-24** Ovarian epithelial inclusion cyst showing cellular atypia (prominent nucleoli, coarse chromatin pattern, nuclear clearing, thickened nuclear membranes). Is this a potential precursor of ovarian cancer? H&E, ×400.

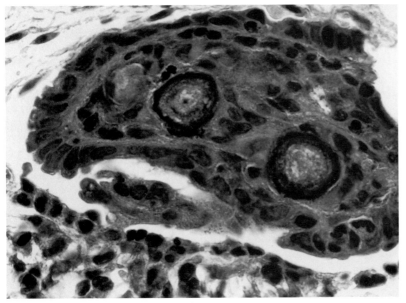

**Fig. 7-25** Peritoneal biopsy from second-look operation for ovarian cancer. Psammoma bodies are surrounded by cells that were interpreted as tumor cells responding to chemotherapy (smaller nuclei than in the primary ovarian carcinoma, paucity of mitoses). H&E, ×400.

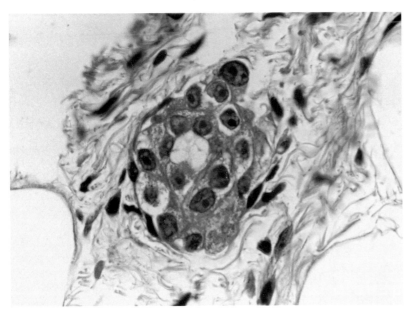

**Fig. 7-26** Peritoneal biopsy from second-look operation for ovarian cancer. Microscopic focus of residual carcinoma, interpreted morphometrically as responsive to chemotherapy. H&E, ×400.

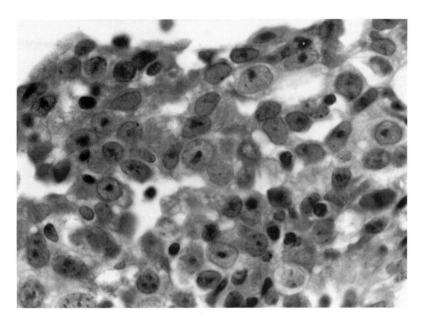

**Fig. 7-27** Peritoneal biopsy from second-look operation for ovarian carcinoma. Computerized image analysis classified the tumor cells as nonresponsive to chemotherapy based on their nuclear profiles. H&E, ×400.

racy to the quantitative diagnostic discriminating power of these rather subtle histologic lesions.[13]

The identification of precursors of ovarian malignancy can also be improved by adding to the morphometric studies, measurements of DNA ploidy, by flow cytometry and immunohistochemistry studies of tumor markers,[14,15] and morphometry of nuclear texture.[16]

Screening programs to benefit the general female population, and especially the population at risk, cannot currently be based on tumor markers in the serum. Tissue diagnosis should be considered as a potentially more reliable method, since the identification of precursors of ovarian and peritoneal malignancy becomes possible with the surgical techniques that make this tissue available. Demonstrating their relationship with invasive cancer, as is the case with dysplastic lesions in other epithelial tissues, should be the object of further studies. The identification of subtle microscopic changes, investigated by objective statistical methods of computerized image analysis, contribute to our insight into the early histogenesis of ovarian cancer.

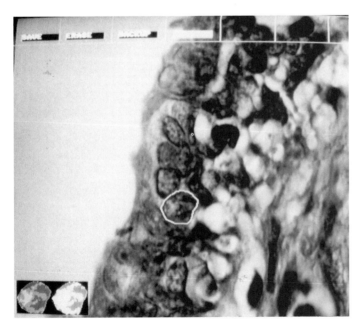

**Fig. 7-28** Ovarian dysplasia: nuclear texture analysis evaluates three levels of gray density (see inset). This method enhances the accuracy of the diagnosis by an objective assessment of the nuclear chromatin.

# REFERENCES

1. Deligdisch L, Gil J. Characterization of ovarian dysplasia by interactive morphometry. *Cancer* 63:748–755, 1989.
2. Plaxe SC, Deligdisch L, Dottino PR, Cohen CJ. Ovarian epithelial neoplasia demonstrated in patients with stage I ovarian carcinoma. *Gynecologic Oncology* 38:367–372, 1990.
3. Gil J, Deligdisch L. Interactive morphometric procedures and statistical analysis in the diagnosis of ovarian dysplasia and carcinoma. *Pathol Res Pract* 185:680–685, 1989.
4. Gusberg SB, Deligdisch L. Ovarian dysplasia. *Cancer* 54:1–4, 1984.
5. Zanaboni F, Accinelli G, Colombo P, Jalmoni G, Morandi C, Pedronetto S. The biological tumor marker's myopia: A model with CA 125 and second look in ovarian cancer. *Int J Biol Markers* 2:105–108, 1987.
6. Cruickshank DJ, Fullerton WT, Klopper A. The clinical significance of pre-operative serum Ca 125 in ovarian cancer. *Br J Obstet Gynecol* 94:692–695, 1987.
7. Laughlan SC. The secondary mullerian system. *Obstet Gynecol Surv* 27:133–146, 1972.
8. Wick MR, Mills SE, Dehner LP, Bollinger DJ, Fechner RE. Serous papillary carcinomas arising from the peritoneum and ovaries. A clinicopathologic and immunohistochemical comparison. *Int J Gynecol Pathol* 8:179–188, 1989.
9. Lindeque BG, Cronje HS, Deale CJ. Prevalence of primary papillary peritoneal neoplasia in patients with ovarian carcinoma. *S Afr Med J* 67:1005–1007, 1985.
10. Feuer GA, Shevchuk KM, Calanog A. Normal sized ovary carcinoma syndrome. *Obstet Gynecol* 73:786–792, 1989.
11. Deligdisch L, Heller D, Gil J. Interactive morphometry of normal and hyperplastic peritoneal mesothelial cells and dysplastic and malignant ovarian cells. *Hum Pathol* 21:218–222, 1990.
12. Deligdisch L, Kerner H, Dargent D, Cohen CJ, Gil J. Morphometric differentiation between responsive tumor cells and mesothelial hyperplasia in second look operation for ovarian cancer. *Hum Pathol* 24:143–147, 1993.
13. Hytiroglou P, Harpaz N, Heller DS, Liu Z, Deligdisch L, Gil J. Differential diagnosis of borderline and invasive serous cystadenocarcinomas of the ovary by computerized interactive morphometric analysis of nuclear features. *Cancer* 69:988–992, 1992.
14. Baak JP. Possibilities and progress of quantitative pathological examination of ovarian tumors. *Eur J Obstet Gynecol Reprod Biol* 29:183–189, 1988.
15. Van Niekerk CC, Boerman OC, Remaekers FC, Poels LG. Marker profile of different phases in the transition of normal human ovarian epithelium to ovarian carcinoma. *Am J Pathol* 138:455–463, 1991.
16. Deligdisch L, Miranda C, Barba J, Gil J. Ovarian Dysplasia: Nuclear Texture Analysis. *Cancer* (in press).

# PART II. PRIMARY NONEPITHELIAL OVARIAN TUMORS

# 8

# Sex Cord–Stromal Tumors

*Vladimir Bychkov, M.D.*

The group of sex cord–stromal tumors includes neoplasms of gonadal epithelial stromal derivation recapitulating in their structure granulosa and theca cells of the ovary or Sertoli and Leydig cells of the testicle. The investigators who believe that all the above-mentioned cell types originate from the specialized stroma of the genital ridge prefer such terms as *mesenchymomas*[1] or *gonadal stromal* tumors.[2] The terms *sex cord–mesenchymal* and *sex cord–stromal* tumors are in line with prevailing view about the epithelial origin of granulosa and Sertoli cells. The last term is adopted in the majority of current publications[3-5] and in the International Histological Classification of Tumors.[6]

Sex cord–stromal tumors constitute about 8% of all ovarian neoplasms.[7-9] They include numerous subtypes as reflected in the WHO classification updated by Young and Scully (Table 8-1).[3]

## GRANULOSA–STROMAL CELL TUMORS

This group includes all tumors consisting of the elements resembling normal ovarian cortex: granulosa, theca, and fibroblasts. They differ significantly in their cellular composition and degree of differentiation but have in common a tendency to produce estrogens. The two main groups are granulosa cell and theca cell tumors, though some neoplasms may contain both elements and are difficult to classify. It is believed that in many such cases the stromal elements are reactive rather than neoplastic. If epithelial elements constitute more than 10% of the mass, the tumors are considered granulosa cell tumors; otherwise they are called thecomas or fibromas with minor sex cord elements.[10]

## GRANULOSA CELL TUMORS

Granulosa cell tumors occur in two distinct forms in different age groups. The most frequent "adult" form is the tumor of middle-aged and older women; the "juvenile" form occurs mostly in children and young adults.

Granulosa cell tumors account for about 1 to 2% of all ovarian neoplasms, with 95% of them of adult type. They are predominantly unilateral. Besides producing symptoms common to ovarian tumors, like low abdominal pain, swelling, etc., they have a tendency to secrete estrogens, causing uterine bleeding due to endometrial hyperplasia, or to produce isosexual precocity in juveniles. On rare occasions androgens are secreted.[11]

Most of the tumors follow a benign course, but at least 10% behave as a low-grade malignancy. The tumor may recur or metastasize for up to 25 years after the initial excision.[12] There is no well-established correlation between the histologic pattern and the clinical behavior, with the exception of the juvenile type of tumor, which displays a more benign course.[13] The factors associated with a relatively poor survival include age over 40, large tumor, bilaterality, extraovarian spread, and numerous mitotic figures.[12]

**Table 8-1**  Classification of Sex Cord–Stromal Tumors

Granulosa–stromal cell tumor
  Granulosa cell tumor
    Adult type
    Juvenile type
  Tumors in the thecoma-fibroma group
    Thecoma
      Typical
      Luteinized
    Fibroma-fibrosarcoma
      Fibroma
      Cellular fibroma
      Fibrosarcoma
  Stromal tumor with minor sex cord elements
  Sclerosing stromal tumor
  Unclassified
Sertoli–stromal cell tumors
  Sertoli cell tumors
  Leydig cell tumor
  Sertoli–Leydig cell tumors
    Well-differentiated
    Of intermediate differentiation
    Poorly differentiated
    With heterologous elements
Gynandroblastoma
Sex cord tumor with annular tubules
Unclassified

### Gross Appearance

Most of the granulosa cell tumors are solid and moderately soft, with areas of cystic degeneration and hemorrhage (Plate 8-1). The solid component is yellow-tan or gray. The gross appearance ranges from predominantly solid to predominantly cystic neoplasms. The latter may be difficult to distinguish from other cystic tumors and nonneoplastic conditions.

### Microscopic Appearance

Granulosa cell tumors display a variety of microscopic patterns, frequently combined in the same neoplasm, making irrelevant an attempt to create a histologic classification of them except for a juvenile type that has its own peculiar pattern.

Microfollicular pattern is the most common in the adult type. It is characterized by the presence of small round cystic spaces, known as the *Call-Exner bodies,* located inside the groups of granulosa-like cells (Fig. 8-1). These spaces are filled with eosinophilic material or contain shrunken nuclei. The cells constituting the bulk of the tumor are round or oval; the cytoplasm is usually scant but may be more conspicuous in case of luteinization. The presence of the nuclei with longitudinal grooves is considered to be typical of this neoplasm (Fig. 8-2).

In the macrofollicular pattern, the cystic structures are lined by granulosa cells in a fashion reminiscent of nonneoplastic cystic follicles (Fig. 8-3), but they lack the well-defined theca interna typical of the latter.

The trabecular pattern is the other classic microscopic representation of the granulosa cell tumor. It is characterized by bands of granulosa cells separated by stroma that may be luteinized (Fig. 8-4). Close to it is the insular form, in which groups of cells are separated by stroma.

The other patterns are represented by the undulated rows, termed "watered silk" (Fig. 8-5), and diffuse

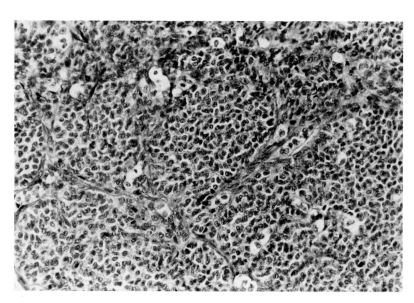

**Fig. 8-1** Granulosa cell tumor, microfollicular type. Small clear spaces containing shrunken nuclei (Call-Exner bodies) are scattered through the tumor. H&E, ×200.

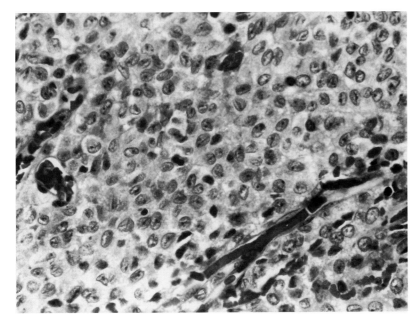

**Fig. 8-2** Granulosa cell tumor. Nuclei are round or oval; some contain longitudinal grooves. H&E, ×450.

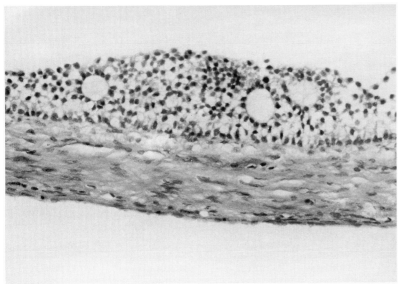

**Fig. 8-3** Granulosa cell tumor with macrofollicular pattern (Note Call-Exner bodies). Thick layer of granulosa and absence of theca interna are evident. H&E, ×200.

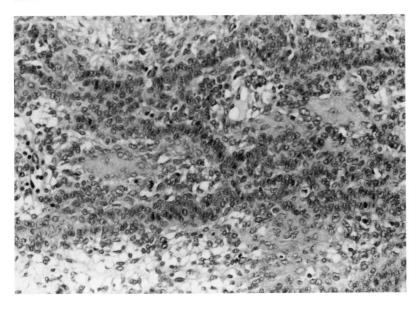

**Fig. 8-4** Granulosa cell tumor with trabecular pattern. Stroma contains cells with clear cytoplasm (luteinization). H&E, ×200.

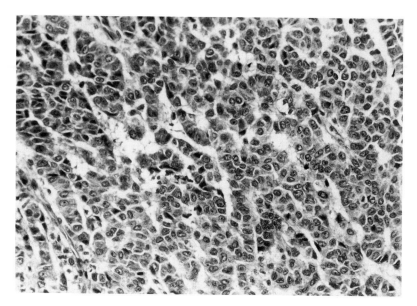

**Fig. 8-5** Granulosa cell tumor composed of undulated rows ("watered silk" pattern). H&E, ×200.

(Fig. 8-6) arrangement of granulosa cells. These two patterns are considered to be less differentiated. Their nuclei are more pleomorphic, the number of mitotic figures is higher, and the nucleoli are more prominent than in other forms.

The juvenile granulosa cell tumors ahve two distinctive features: they show solid arrangement with the presence of small follicles (Fig. 8-7) and the cells have well-developed eosinophilic or clear cytoplasm typical of luteinization (Fig. 8-8). Their nuclei are more pleomorphic than those of the adult type of tumors and lack grooving.

Enzyme histochemistry and electron microscopy in-

dicate that granulosa cells take a very small part in estrogen production, and that the bulk of this activity falls on the theca cells in the stroma.[14]

Immunohistochemical studies reveal significant positivity for vimentin, isolated cytokeratin-positive cells, and lack of carcinoembryonic antigen in granulosa cell tumors.[13]

### Differential Diagnosis

Granulosa cell tumors have to be differentiated from common carcinomas, small cell carcinoma, carcinoid, and Sertoli-cell tumor. Unlike cells of common carci-

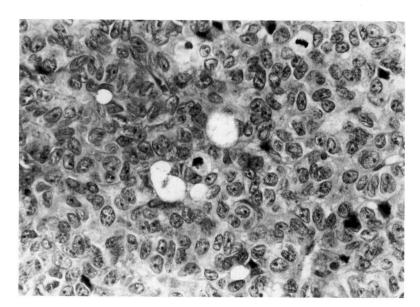

**Fig. 8-6** Granulosa cell tumor with diffuse pattern. Notice pleomorphic nuclei, prominent nucleoli, and mitotic figures. H&E, ×450.

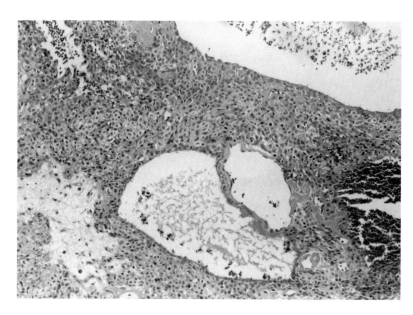

**Fig. 8-7** Juvenile granulosa cell tumor characterized by the solid arrangement of luteinized cells and by the presence of small follicules. H&E, ×150.

noma, the cells of granulosa cell tumor are much less pleomorphic, have grooved nuclei, and are arranged in a better-organized fashion. In a case of poorly differentiated granulosa cell tumor, a staining reaction for peanut agglutinin (PNA) may be helpful because of PNA positivity of common epithelial tumors versus PNA negativity of granulosa cell tumors.[15] Small cell carcinomas have very bizarre cellular composition and much higher mitotic rate than any granulosa cell tumors. Differentiation with carcinoids may present a serious difficulty, but their immunohistochemical reaction with neuroendocrine markers solves the problem. Sertoli cell tumors have well-outlined tubules, but some poorly differentiated types may be indistinguishable from the granulosa

cell tumors and thus fall into the category of unclassified sex cord stromal tumors.

## THECOMA

Thecomas are two times less frequent than granulosa cell tumors and are mostly encountered in older age groups. The majority of the patients are postmenopausal, with a mean age of 59 years.[16] The tumors are unilateral in 97% of the cases and almost always follow a benign course. Most of them produce estrogens, and the main clinical symptom is uterine bleeding after menopause. A few luteinized thecomas display an androgenic effect.[3]

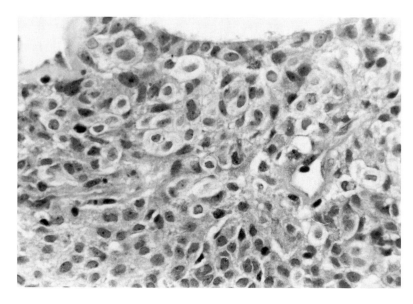

**Fig. 8-8** Juvenile granulosa cell tumor showing luteinization. Notice the absence of grooved nuclei. H&E, ×450.

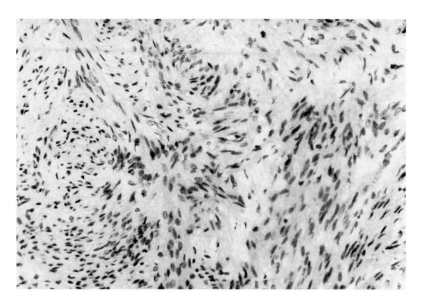

**Fig. 8-9** Theca cell tumor. Classic pattern consisting of interlacing bundles of elongated stromal cells. H&E, ×250.

*Gross Appearance*

Thecomas are predominantly solid tumors with characteristic yellow discoloration plate (Plate 8-2). They may be also whitish-gray with focal yellow streaks. They usually do not exceed 10 cm in diameter.

*Microscopic Appearance*

The tumors consist of oval or elongated cells forming poorly delineated bundles creating a pattern similar to that of normal cortical stroma (Fig. 8-9). Many thecomas contain cells with well-developed clear or eosinophilic cytoplasm (Fig. 8-10). These tumors are sometimes referred to as "luteinized" thecomas.

Mitotic figures are rare, but some thecomas may be very cellular and show enhanced mitotic activity (Fig. 8-11). A few of those follow a malignant course, usually by continuous growth rather than by metastatic spread.

Lipid staining is usually positive, and polarizing microscopy reveals numerous anisotropic droplets.

## FIBROMA

Fibromas are the most frequent among sex cord–stromal tumors and account for 4% of all ovarian neoplasms. The average age of a patient with fibroma is 48 years.[17] Bilateral tumors occur in less than 10% of the cases.

Fibromas do not produce steroid hormones. They may be associated with ascites and hydrothorax

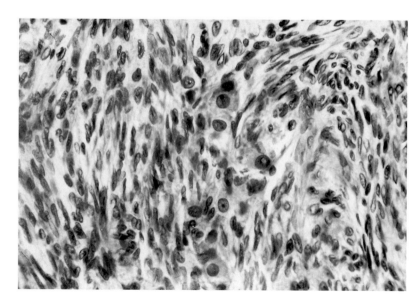

**Fig. 8-10** Theca cell tumor containing plump cells with round nuclei and well-developed cytoplasm (luteinization). H&E, ×450.

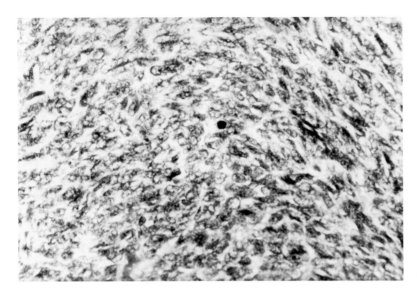

**Fig. 8-11** Cellular thecoma containing mitotic figures. H&E, ×450.

(Meigs's syndrome) that disappear after removal of the tumor.[18] They are benign in 100% of the cases, and the rare malignant counterpart warrants the designation of fibrosarcoma.[19]

### Gross Appearance

Fibromas vary significantly in size. Many of them are quite small. According to Young and Scully, the nodules less than 3 cm in diameter should not be considered true neoplasms.[3] They are hard and reveal chalky-white whorled appearance on cross-section. Foci of calcification may be present.

### Microscopic Appearance

Fibromas consist of slender elongated cells depositing collagen. Whorly appearance of collagen bundles is the same as in fibromas at other locations, but edema is a frequent peculiar finding in ovarian fibromas (Fig. 8-12). An admixture of tubular epithelial structures accounting for less than 10% of the tumor mass has no clinical implications (Fig. 8-13), and these tumors are termed *fibromas with minor sex cord elements*.[10]

Nuclear atypia and mitoses are very rare in fibromas. The presence of more than four mitotic figures per 10 high-power fields is suggestive of a malignant course.[20]

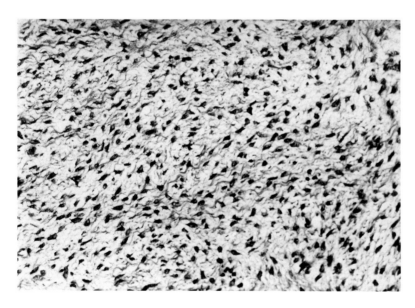

**Fig. 8-12** Fibroma with edematous stroma. H&E, ×200.

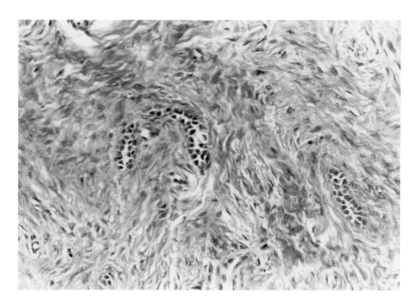

**Fig. 8-13** Fibroma with minor sex cord elements. H&E, ×250.

## SCLEROSING STROMAL TUMOR

Sclerosing stromal tumor was described as a distinct entity in 1973 by Chalvardjian and Scully.[21] It differs from thecoma and fibroma by occurring mostly in the first three decades of life, and by contrast to thecoma it very rarely secretes estrogens. The tumor is always unilateral and benign.

### Gross Appearance

Sclerosing stromal tumor is a discrete, sharply demarcated mass buried under ovarian surface. Its surface is solid and white and often shows edema, cyst formation, and areas of yellow discoloration.

### Microscopic Appearance

The tumor consists of moderately cellular areas alternating with thick collagen bundles. Groups of cells with vacuolated cytoplasm and numerous thin-walled dilated vessels create a characteristic picture (Fig. 8-14).

## SERTOLI–STROMAL CELL TUMORS

Sertoli–stromal cell tumors, also known as *androblastomas* and *arrhenoblastomas*, are rare and constitute only 1% of all sex cord–stromal tumors of the ovaries.[4] They include neoplasms with variable histologic patterns characterized by the presence of Sertoli-like and Leydig-

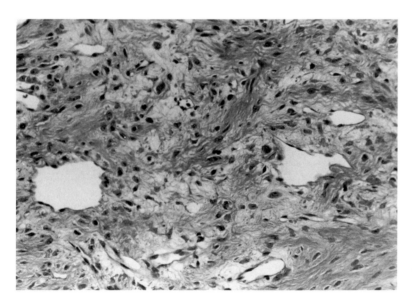

**Fig. 8-14** Sclerosing stromal tumor containing thin-walled vessels and cells with clear cytoplasm. H&E, ×250.

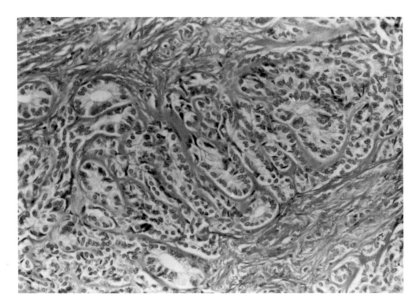

**Fig. 8-15** Sertoli cell tumor. Tubular structures lined by columnar epithelial cells are seen. H&E, ×250.

like elements in different combinations and with different degrees of differentiation. Three categories of them, based on their histologic pattern and clinical presentation, merit separate description: pure Sertoli cell, pure Leydig cell, and combined Sertoli–Leydig cell tumor.

## SERTOLI CELL TUMOR

The Sertoli cell tumor, which is benign and unilateral, accounts for about 4% of Sertoli–stromal cell tumors. Unlike other tumors in this category that produce androgens, it tends to produce estrogens and may cause isosexual precocity.[3]

### Gross Appearance

Sertoli cell tumor averages approximately 9 cm in diameter and forms a solid, lobulated, yellow or brown mass.

### Microscopic Appearance

The tumor consists of hollow tubules lined by columnar epithelium oriented toward basement membrane (Fig. 8-15), hence the alternative term *tubular androblastoma*. Some tumors contain lipid droplets in the cytoplasm. Mitoses are rarely seen. The stroma is fibrotic and devoid of Leydig cells.

### Differential Diagnosis

By virtue of its resemblance to glandular tissue, Sertoli cell tumor may present a serious diagnostic problem.

Absence of secretions in the glands makes it different from the majority of the common epithelial tumors. The other helpful feature is the lack of PNA lectin binding in Sertoli cell tumor, while common epithelial neoplasms are PNA-positive.[15]

Krukenberg tumor may show some resemblance to Sertoli cell tumor, but it is usually bilateral and mucin-positive.

Differentiation from carcinoid may be based on the Sertoli cell tumor's positive immunohistochemical reaction with neuron-specific enolase and other neurosecretory markers.

## LEYDIG CELL TUMOR

Leydig cell tumors are usually small and originate in the ovarian hilus, hence the synonym *hilus cell tumor*. The ages of the patients are higher than in other Sertoli–stromal cell tumors, with an average of 58 years. The tumor produces virilization in about 75% of the patients.[22] Practically all pure Leydig cell tumors are benign.

### Gross Appearance

The tumor is usually solid, reddish-brown, or yellow.

### Microscopic Appearance

The tumor consists of a closely packed mass of large polyhedral cells with eosinophilic cytoplasm and round nuclei (Fig. 8-16). The hallmark of the tumor is the presence of crystals of Reincke, rectangular or rodlike

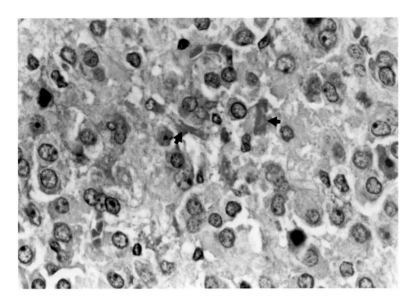

**Fig. 8-16** Leydig cell tumor. Solid arrangement of polyhedral cells, some containing crystals of Reincke (indicated by arrows), is characteristic. H&E, ×450.

cytoplasmic structures surrounded by a halo. They are found, however, in only 50% of the cases. Even in their absence, a classic histologic picture and a location in the hilus make the diagnosis easy.

## SERTOLI–LEYDIG CELL TUMORS

Sertoli–Leydig cell tumors constitute the majority of the Sertoli–stromal cell group and are mostly seen at younger ages, with 75% of the patients below 30 years.[3] The most characteristic mode of clinical presentation is virilization, but it happens in only one-third of the patients. The other symptoms are common to all ovarian tumors. Almost all the tumors are unilateral.

Prognosis depends in significant degree on microscopic appearance. Well-differentiated tumors show persistently benign behavior, tumors with intermediate differentiation have unfavorable prognosis in 11%, and poorly differentiated tumors are malignant in 59% of the cases.

### Gross Appearance

Sertoli–Leydig cell tumors may reach up to 15 cm in diameter and grossly resemble granulosa cell tumors with the exception of the cystic form of the latter, which is not encountered among them.

### Microscopic Appearance

There are many microscopic patterns seen in the Sertoli–Leydig cell tumors, allowing their histologic grading as reflected in the WHO classification (see Table 8-1).

The well-differentiated tumors are characterized by a tubular pattern similar to one seen in pure Sertoli cell tumors combined with clusters of Leydig-type cells in the stroma (Fig. 8-17). The latter are polyhedral and have well-developed eosinophilic or clear cytoplasm and centrally located round nuclei. They may contain crystals of Reincke.

The intermediate pattern consists of closely packed and less differentiated tubules lined by multilayered epithelium (Fig. 8-18). Mitotic figures may be seen. Luteinized cells of Leydig type are clearly visible in the stroma. Further dedifferentiation is characterized by the disappearance of the luminal pattern and by the replacement of the tubular component by the trabecular structures (Fig. 8-19).

Arrangement of tubular structures in a pattern reminiscent of rete testis (Fig. 8-20) earned these tumors the name *retiform*. The retiform tumors are seen at the youngest ages in this group, are almost never virilizing, and show malignant behavior in about one-third of the cases.[23]

Some Sertoli–Leydig cell tumors contain heterologous elements consisting of intestinal-type inclusions, elements of carcinoid, cartilage, and even rhabdomyosarcoma. The heterologous elements are considered to be prognostically unfavorable.

Poorly differentiated Sertoli cell tumors display a predominantly sarcomatoid pattern consisting of densely packed elongated and oval cells with a focal tendency to form poorly outlined tubular structures (Fig. 8-21).

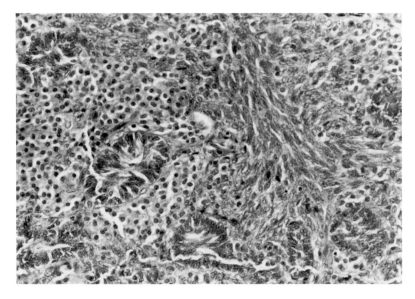

**Fig. 8-17** Sertoli–Leydig cell tumors, well differentiated. Stroma contains Leydig cells. H&E, ×200.

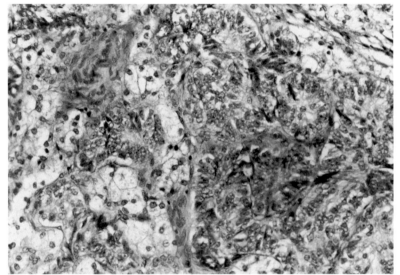

**Fig. 8-18** Sertoli–Leydig cell tumor of intermediate differentiation. Tubular structures are closely packed and lined by multilayered epithelium. H&E, ×200.

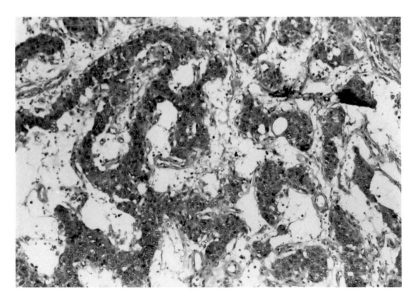

**Fig. 8-19** Sertoli–Leydig cell tumor of intermediate to poor differentiation displaying trabecular pattern. H&E, ×150.

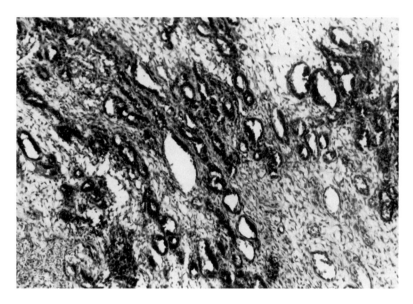

**Fig. 8-20** Sertoli–Leydig cell tumor with retiform pattern. H&E, × 100.

### Differential Diagnosis

The great variety of patterns in Sertoli–Leydig cell tumors may present some diagnostic problems. Those that contain Leydig cells are easier to differentiate.

The tumors with a predominant retiform pattern are the ones most frequently confused with the common epithelial type of carcinoma. Negative PNA lectin binding versus positive binding in common epithelial tumors may be helpful.

## GYNANDROBLASTOMA

Gynandroblastoma, which is extremely rare, should contain a significant proportion of both Sertoli and granulosa cell components to warrant its name (Fig. 8-22). A less than 10% presence of one of the components implies that the tumor belongs to either the granulosa cell or the Sertoli cell group.

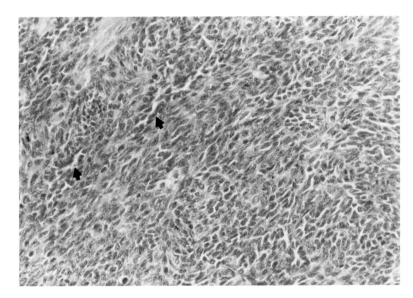

**Fig. 8-21** Poorly differentiated Sertoli–Leydig cell tumor with sarcomatoid pattern. Poorly outlined tubular structures (indicated by arrows) are being formed locally.

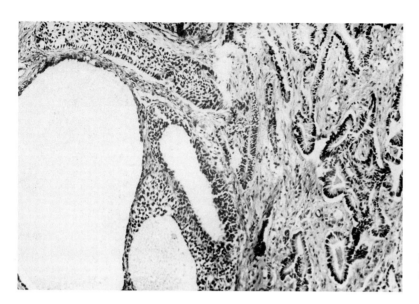

**Fig. 8-22** Gynandroblastoma. Tubular structures are seen together with follicular elements. H&E, ×100.

## SEX CORD TUMORS WITH ANNULAR TUBULES

There are two distinct patterns of presentation of the sex chord tumor with annular tubules. One-third of them occur in women with the Peutz-Jeghers syn-

The few cases reported in the literature mention solid, pale tumors less than 6 cm in diameter.[24]

drome. They are usually bilateral, calcified, and very small.[25] The others, unassociated with Peutz-Jeghers syndrome, are relatively large and unilateral, with 20% pursuing a malignant course.[26] The mean age of the patients is 27 years for the first type, and 34 years for the second.

The microscopic hallmark is the presence of concentric structures containing rows of epithelial cells concentrated around the periphery and around a hyalinized material located in the center of the concentric tubule (Fig. 8-23).

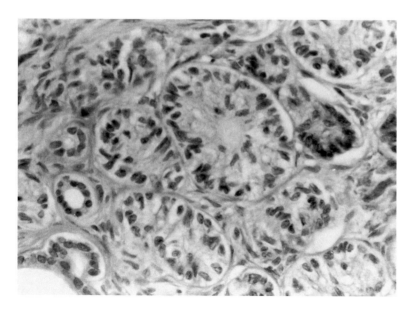

**Fig. 8-23** Sex cord tumor with annular tubules. H&E, ×200.

## PLATES

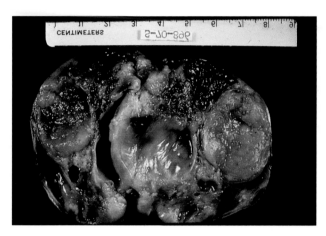

**Plate 8-1.** Granulosa cell tumor with areas of cystic degeneration and hemorrhage.

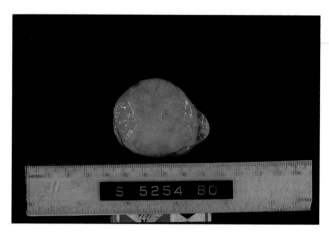

**Plate 8-2.** Theca cell tumor. Note yellow discoloration.

# REFERENCES

1. Busby T, Anderson GW. Feminizing mesenchymomas of the ovary. *Am J Obstet Gynecol* 68:1391–1399, 1954.

2. Novak ER, Kutchmeshgi J, Mupas RS, Woodruff JD. Feminizing gonadal stromal tumors. *Obstet Gynecol* 38:701–712, 1971.

3. Young RH, Scully RE. Sex cord–stromal, steroid cell, and other ovarian tumors with endocrine, paraendocrine, and paraneoplastic manifestations. In *Blaustein's Pathology of the Female Genital Tract,* 3d ed, Kurman RJ, ed. New York, Springer-Verlag, 1987, pp 607–646.

4. Russell P, Bannatyne P. *Surgical Pathology of the Ovaries.* Edinburgh, Churchill Livingstone, 1989, pp 316–378.

5. Roth LM. Sex cord–stromal and lipid cell tumours of the ovaries. In *Hains and Taylor Obstetrical and Gynecological Pathology,* Fox H, ed. Edinburgh, Churchill Livingstone, 1987, vol. 1, pp 624–636.

6. Serov SF, Scully RE, Sobin LH. *Histological Typing of Ovarian Tumors.* International Histological Classification of Tumors, no. 9. Geneva, World Health Organization, 1973.

7. Bennington JL, Ferguson BR, Haber SL. Incidence and relative frequency of benign and malignant ovarian neoplasms. *Obstet Gynecol* 32:627–732, 1968.

8. Gee DC, Russell P. The pathological assessment of ovarian neoplasms: IV. The sex cord stromal tumors. *Pathology* 13:235–255, 1981.

9. Yaker A, Benirschke K. A ten year study of ovarian tumors. *Virchows Arch [Pathol Anat]* 366:275–286, 1975.

10. Young RH, Scully RE. Ovarian stromal tumors with minor sex cord elements. *Int J Gynaecol Pathol* 2:227–232, 1983.

11. Jarabak J, Talerman A. Virilization due to metastasizing granulosa cell tumor. *Int J Gynecol Pathol* 2:316–324, 1983.

12. Fox H, Agrawal K, Langley FA. A clinicopathologic study of 92 cases of granulosa cell tumor of the ovary with special reference to the factors influencing prognosis. *Cancer* 35:231–241, 1975.

13. Biscotti CV, Hart WR. Juvenile granulosa cell tumors of the ovary. *Arch Pathol Lab Med* 113:40–46, 1989.

14. Woodruff JD, Williams TJ, Goldberg B, Lauterbach M, Preece E. Hormonal activity of the common ovarian neoplasms. *Am J Obstet Gynecol* 87:679–691, 1973.

15. Bychkov V, Deligdisch L, Talerman A, et al. Lectin histochemistry of sex cord–stromal tumors and small cell carcinoma of the ovaries. *Gynecol Obstet Invest,* 34:715–718, 1992.

16. Bjorkholm E, Silversward C. Theca-cell tumors. Clinical features and prognosis. *Acta Radiol Oncol Radiat Phys Biol* 19:241–250, 1980.

17. Morrison CW, Woodruff JD. Fibrothecoma and associated ovarian stromal neoplasia. *Obstet Gynecol* 23:344–349, 1964.

18. Meigs JV. Fibroma of the ovary with ascites and hydrothorax. *Am J Obstet Gynecol* 67:962–968, 1954.

19. Prat J, Scully RE. Cellular fibromas and fibrosarcomas of the ovary. *Cancer* 47:2663–2669, 1981.

20. Miles PA, Kiley KC, Mena H. Giant fibrosarcoma of the ovary. *Int J Gynecol Pathol* 4:83–87, 1985.

21. Chalvardjian A, Scully RE. Sclerosing stromal tumors of the ovary. *Cancer* 31:664–668, 1973.

22. Dunnihoo DR, Grieme DL, Woolf RB. Hilar-cell tumors of the ovary. *Obstet Gynecol* 27:703–709, 1966.

23. Talerman A. Ovarian Sertoli–Leydig cell tumor (androblastoma) with retiform pattern. *Cancer* 60:3056–3064, 1987.

24. Jaworski R, Fryatt JI, Turner TB, et al. Gynandroblastoma of the ovary. *Pathology* 18:348–351, 1986.

25. Young RH, Welch WR, Dickersin GR, et al. Ovarian sex cord tumor with annular tubules. *Cancer* 50:1384–1402, 1982.

26. Fox H. Sex cord–stromal tumors of the ovary. *J Pathol* 145:127–148, 1985.

# 9

# Germ Cell Tumors

*Tamara Kalir, M.D., Ph.D.*

The ovarian germ cell tumors are oocyte-derived, in contrast to tumors of ovarian epithelial, sex cord, or stromal cell origin. Of adult ovarian neoplasms, epithelial tumors are the most common. Germ cell tumors rank second and comprise almost one-quarter of ovarian neoplasms.[1] Most adult germ cell tumors are benign and are mature cystic teratomas. In contrast, in children and adolescents, both benign and malignant germ cell tumors constitute a greater proportion of ovarian neoplasms.[2]

The various germ cell tumors, their histogenesis, and their level of differentiation are shown in Fig. 9-1. Many of these ovarian neoplasms are more likely to occur in mixed germ cell tumors than in pure form.

## DYSGERMINOMA

Dysgerminomas occur in patients of all ages, but are most frequent in women under 30.[3] Although they constitute less than 2% of all ovarian neoplasms, dysgerminomas are the most common of the malignant germ cell tumors.[3] The cells are malignant primordial, or undifferentiated, oocytes arrested at a point prior to meiotic division—they contain twice the amount of DNA as in normal diploid cells[4]—and prior to sexual differentiation—*dys* from *dis,* meaning "two," referring to the sexes.[5]

### GROSS

The tumors are usually unilateral and favor the right ovary.[6] They are ovoid-encapsulated masses, ranging from 3 to 50 cm.[4] Consistency varies from firm to soft, the latter in larger tumors with extensive necrosis. The cut surface is solid, homogeneous, and gray, tan, or pink (Fig. 9-2). Areas of hemorrhage may be seen. Cystic spaces are the result either of necrosis or of the presence of other neoplastic germ cell elements.

## HISTOLOGY

Tumor cells are arranged in either diffuse masses, smaller islands, or columns with intervening sparse to abundantly fibrous stroma, which characteristically contains lymphocytes and occasionally, granulomata, eosinophils, or plasma cells (Fig. 9-3).

Tumor cells are large and monomorphic, distinctly round or polygonal, with pale eosinophilic or clear cytoplasm. Nuclei are central, with one or more prominent nucleoli. Chromatin is vesicular or uneven finely granular. Mitotic activity is variable.

## ENDODERMAL SINUS (YOLK SAC) TUMOR

Endodermal sinus tumor occurs in patients of all ages, but is most common in those under 20.[7] It is the second most common malignant ovarian germ cell tumor, after dysgerminoma, to occur in pure form and is the most common highly-malignant germ cell neoplasm.[8] Endodermal sinus tumor also occurs in combination with other neoplastic germ cell elements. It is a malignant derivative of yolk sac endoderm.

147

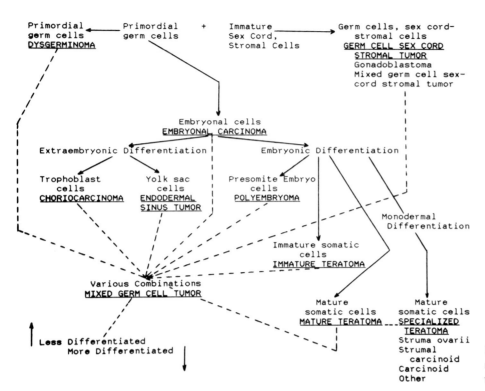

**Fig. 9-1** The ovarian germ cell tumors: histogenesis and level of differentiation.

## GROSS

Endodermal sinus tumors generally are unilateral and favor the right ovary. They are round, smooth-surfaced tumors, ranging from 7 to 28 cm.[7] Consistency varies from firm to gelatinous. Cut surface is semisolid and pink or gray, with hemorrhagic, necrotic, and cystic areas.

## HISTOLOGY

Endodermal sinus tumors characteristically exhibit a wide range of patterns, many of which can occur in the same tumor. Some patterns (including microcystic, alveolar-glandular, polyvesicular-vitelline, myxomatous, and macrocystic) show cysts, microcysts, irregular cavities, or glandular spaces in a loose myxoid or

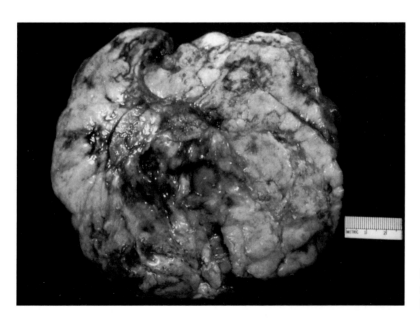

**Fig. 9-2** Dysgerminoma. Cut surface is solid and gray, with several areas of hemorrhage and necrosis.

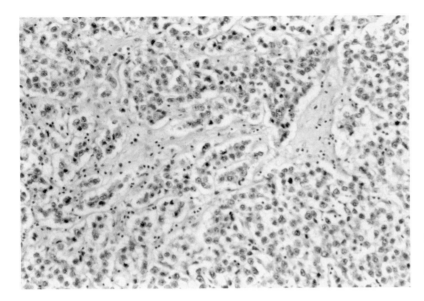

**Fig. 9-3** Dysgerminoma showing large aggregates of neoplastic cells and intervening fibrous septae containing lymphocytes. H&E, ×200.

compact stroma. Other patterns include papillary structures (papillary pattern) or Schiller-Duval bodies (endodermal sinus pattern) (Fig.9-4). The latter structures are diagnostic of endodermal sinus tumor and resemble the endodermal sinuses of the rat placenta (Fig. 9-5). They consist of a central fibrovascular core lined by epithelial-like cells, which may project into a capsular space. Other patterns (solid, hepatoid, primitive endodermal) show solid aggregates of tumor cells. The primitive endodermal pattern can additionally show gland formation.

Tumor cells lining cysts and cavities vary from flat to cuboidal, columnar, or mucinous epithelial. Solid patterns contain polygonal tumor cells with clear or eosinophilic cytoplasm. Nuclei are large and hyperchromatic, or vesicular with prominent nucleoli. Mitotic activity is usually brisk. Small intra- or extracellular eosinophilic globules that contain AFP, $\alpha_1$-antitrypsin, or transferrin may be present. Similar globules are found in other poorly differentiated neoplasms and are not specific for endodermal sinus tumor.[1]

## EMBRYONAL CARCINOMA

Embryonal carcinomas occur in children and adults under age 30[9] and are highly malignant. They are uncom-

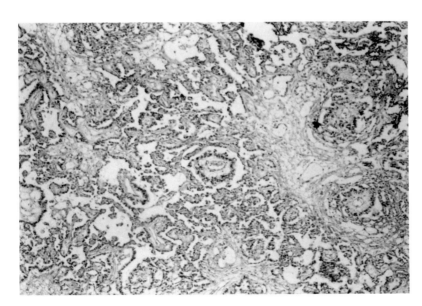

**Fig. 9-4** Endodermal sinus tumor, showing endodermal sinus pattern, with Schiller-Duval bodies, in both longitudinal and transverse section. H&E, ×80.

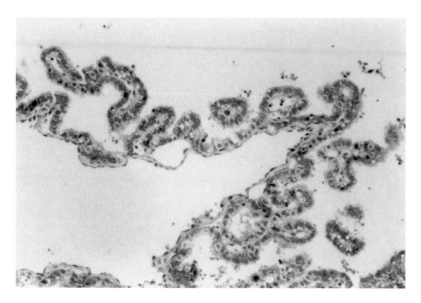

**Fig. 9-5** Rat placenta, showing endodermal sinuses, in longitudinal and transverse section, containing nucleated red blood cells. H&E, ×200.

mon and are more likely to be seen in mixed germ cell tumors than in pure form. The tumor is composed of undifferentiated neoplastic embryonal cells, capable of very early differentiation into extraembryonic as well as embryonic structures.

## GROSS

Since embryonal carcinomas usually occur in mixed germ cell tumors, appearances vary depending on the amount and type of germ cell elements present. Areas containing embryonal carcinoma are solid and gray or white, with patches of hemorrhage and necrosis.

## HISTOLOGY

Embryonal carcinomas range from completely undifferentiated, in which cells grow as solid aggregates, to better differentiated, in which clefts, glands, or papillary structures are seen reminiscent of very primitive embryonic or yolk sac elements. Primitive mesenchymal tissue may be present (Fig. 9-6).

Tumor cells are medium to large ovoid or, in better-differentiated tumors, columnar with abundant pale eosinophilic cytoplasm and ill-defined plasma membranes. Nuclei are central, large, and sharply defined. Chromatin is dark or vesicular with one or more nucleoli. Giant cells and multinucleated cells, including

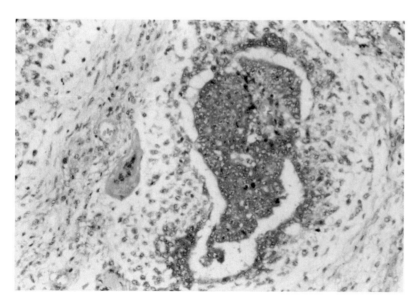

**Fig. 9-6** Embryonal carcinoma, showing solid aggregate of neoplastic embryonal cells and surrounding loose mesenchyme containing syncytiotrophoblast. H&E, ×200.

syncytiotrophoblasts, may be seen. Mitotic activity is brisk. Primitive yolk sac elements may synthesize AFP.[9] Syncytiotrophoblasts may produce chorionic gonadotropin and placental lactogen.[10]

## POLYEMBRYOMA

Polyembryomas are highly malignant and occur in girls and young adults.[11] They are more often seen in mixed germ cell tumors than in pure form. They derive from embryonal cells that have differentiated into structures resembling presomite embryos.[12]

### GROSS

Polyembryomas are usually unilateral and range from 9.5[12] to 34 cm.[11] Cut surface is solid and pink or gray with areas of hemorrhage.

### HISTOLOGY

Tumors contain numerous embryoid bodies haphazardly arranged in a collagenous stroma (Fig. 9-7). The embryoid bodies vary in size and developmental stage from primitive to well-formed to malformed. Well-formed embryoids show an embryonic disc, yolk sac, and amniotic cavity. The embryonic disc is two-sided: the yolk sac side is composed of uniform cuboidal, endoderm-like cells; the amniotic side is composed of tall, columnar, ectoderm-like cells. The surrounding mesenchyme may contain syncytiotrophoblasts.[12] The extraembryonic elements can produce AFP, chorionic gonadotropin, and placental lactogen.[12,13]

## CHORIOCARCINOMA

The majority of patients with primary ovarian choriocarcinoma are under 20 years old. These neoplasms are very rare and are more likely to be found in mixed germ cell tumors than in pure form.[14] They are highly malignant and composed of neoplastic trophoblast cells.

### GROSS

Areas in mixed germ cell tumors containing choriocarcinoma are solid but friable, and gray or white with hemorrhage and necrosis.

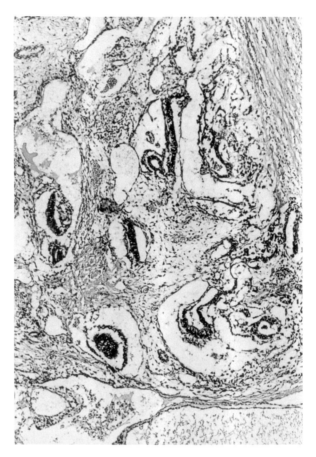

**Fig. 9-7** Polyembryoma, showing multiple embryoid bodies in collagenous stroma. H&E, ×125. (Courtesy Professor J. Ringsted, Odense, Denmark.)

### HISTOLOGY

Choriocarcinomas are composed of masses of malignant cyto- and syncytiotrophoblasts surrounded by hemorrhage. Stroma is absent. There is great variation in the pattern and amount of the two cell types (Fig. 9-8).

Cytotrophoplasts are medium-sized, round or polygonal cells with amphophilic or clear cytoplasm. Nuclei are central, small, and hyperchromatic, or large and vesicular. Nuclear membranes and nucleoli are prominent. Mitotic activity is brisk. Syncytiotrophoblasts are large, basophilic vacuolated cells containing multiple hyperchromatic nuclei that vary in size and shape. Mitotic figures are absent. The cells secrete chorionic gonadotropin and placental lactogen.[10,11]

## IMMATURE TERATOMA

Immature, or malignant, teratomas are rare. They usually occur in patients under age 20.[15] The tumors are

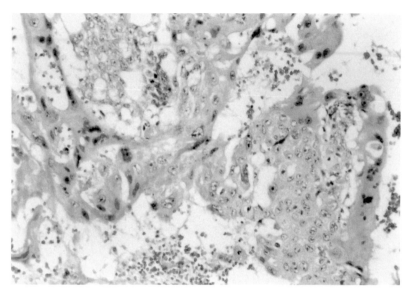

**Fig. 9-8** Choriocarcinoma, showing neoplastic syncytiotrophoblast (peripheral, multinucleated) and cytotrophoblast cells (central). H&E, ×200.

composed of immature or fetal and, frequently, mature tissues derived from the three germ layers.

## GROSS

Immature teratomas are usually unilateral oval masses that range from 7 to 28 cm.[16] Consistency varies from soft to firm. Cut surface is solid gray or dark brown, with some cystic areas. Foci containing cartilage or bone may be seen.

## HISTOLOGY

The tumors contain tissues derived from the three germ layers, haphazardly arranged, and varying in state of differentiation from immature to mature. Neuroectoderm usually predominates and may take the form of glia or neuroepithelial rosettes and tubules (Fig. 9-9). Mitotic activity is variable. Poorly differentiated tumors contain more immature tissue.[17]

## MATURE TERATOMA

Mature teratomas occur in patients of all ages, but are commonly seen in women in their reproductive years. Mature cystic teratoma (dermoid) is the most common ovarian teratoma and the most common ovarian germ cell neoplasm. The tumors are thought to arise from oocytes by parthenogenesis.[18] They are composed of

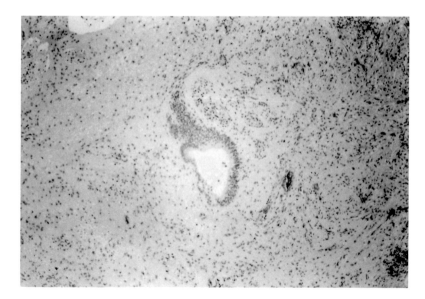

**Fig. 9-9** Immature teratoma, showing immature neural tissue containing glial cells and neuroepithelial structure, reminiscent of neural tube. H&E, ×200.

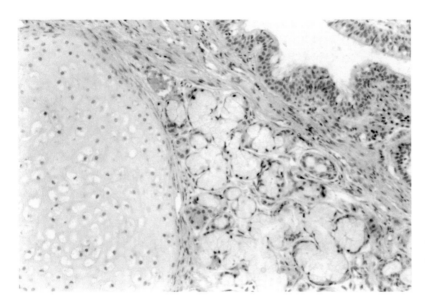

**Fig. 9-10** Mature teratoma, showing fully differentiated tissue composed of respiratory epithelium, cartilage, and seromucinous glands, reminiscent of bronchus. H&E, ×200.

fully differentiated tissues derived from the three germ layers, with ectoderm predominating. Mature teratomatous tissue may be present, with other neoplastic elements, in mixed germ cell tumors. In rare cases, usually of postmenopausal women, mature teratomas undergo malignant transformation.[15]

### GROSS

(Plate 9-1). The tumors generally are unilateral ovoid, cystic masses ranging in size from 0.5 to 45 cm.[19] Consistency is soft and gelatinous with some firm areas. Cut surface shows one or more cysts that contain yellow sebaceous material and hair. Partially developed organs or portions of organ systems may be recognizable. Rokitansky's protuberance, or dermoid mamilla, may be identified in one or more areas as a nodular or polypoid mass that may contain bone or teeth.

### HISTOLOGY

Mature teratomas show fully differentiated tissues arranged in an organized fashion: ciliated respiratory epithelium usually overlies cartilage (Fig. 9-10) and adjacent minor salivary glands, reminiscent of bronchus. Most cysts are lined by keratinized epidermis with underlying hair follicles and sebaceous and sweat glands. Surrounding ovarian stroma may be fibrotic and contain foreign body giant cells.

## MONODERMAL (SPECIALIZED) TERATOMAS

Monodermal teratomas are thought to result from one-sided development in a mature teratoma.

## STRUMA OVARII

Struma ovarii constitutes 2.7% of ovarian teratomas.[20] The majority of patients are in their reproductive years. The term applies to tumors in which thyroid tissue is either the sole or the predominant component, or is grossly recognizable. Very rarely, the tumors are malignant.[21]

### GROSS

(Plate 9-2). Struma ovarii is usually unilateral and smaller than 10 cm in diameter. Cut surface is tan and glistening and may show small yellow or brown cystic spaces containing colloid.

### HISTOLOGY

The tumor resembles mature thyroid tissue and consists of differently sized colloid-containing acini lined by columnar or flattened epithelium.

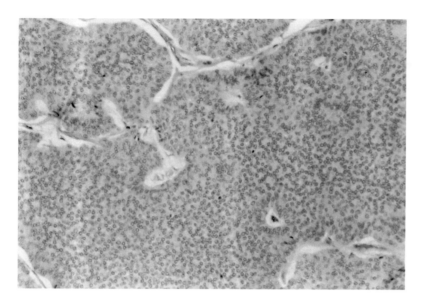

**Fig. 9-11** Carcinoid, insular, showing solid sheets of monomorphic tumor cells and intervening delicate fibrovascular network. H&E, ×200.

## CARCINOID

Carcinoids may be pure or associated with other mature teratomatous components. There are four types: insular (most common), trabecular, mucinous, and strumal. Patients with carcinoid are commonly peri- or postmenopausal. The tumors arise from ovarian argentaffin or enterochromaffin cells.

### GROSS

Tumors generally are unilateral and firm, ranging in size from microscopic to 25 cm.[1] Cut surface is solid, homogeneous tan or yellow.

## HISTOLOGY

Tumor cells are arranged either in acini and solid nests (insular (Fig. 9-11) and mucinous types) or thin, parallel-running ribbons (trabecular type) (Fig. 9-12). Surrounding stroma ranges from loose to densely fibrous. Mucinous carcinoids may also contain larger cysts and pools of extracellular mucin. The cells are uniformly polygonal, cuboidal, or columnar with generous basophilic or amphophilic cytoplasm containing orange-brown argentaffin or argyrophil granules. Nuclei are central and round, with dark or stippled chromatin and prominent nucleoli. Mucinous carcinoids also contain intraglandular goblet cells and infiltrating signet ring cells (Fig. 9-13). Mitotic activity is low. Strumal carci-

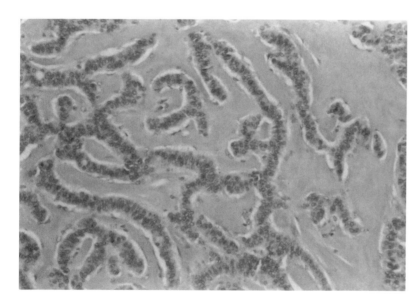

**Fig. 9-12** Carcinoid, trabecular, showing parallel-running cords of tumor cells in hyalinized stroma. H&E, ×200.

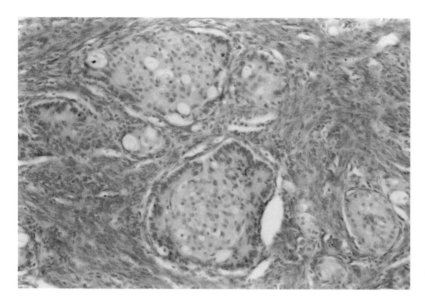

**Fig. 9-13** Carcinoid, mucinous, showing tumor cell nests with cystic spaces containing mucin. H&E, ×80.

noid is composed of colloid-filled follicles of thyroid tissue adjacent to, or admixed with, trabecular or insular carcinoid (Fig. 9-14).

## OTHER MONODERMAL TERATOMAS

Included in this category are such tumors as epidermoid cyst, sebaceous gland tumor, malignant neuroectodermal tumors, and, possibly, gastrointestinal-type mucinous tumors.

## GERM CELL-SEX CORD–STROMAL TUMORS

Germ cell sex cord–stromal tumors are composed of primordial germ cells admixed with immature sex cord and stromal cells. There are two types: gonadoblastoma and mixed germ cell-sex cord–stromal tumor. Both types of tumor can occur in pure form or in association with other malignant germ cell elements.

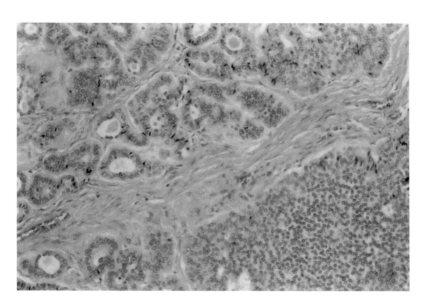

**Fig. 9-14** Carcinoid, strumal, showing thyroid tissue (top) merging with trabecular carcinoid (bottom). H&E, ×80.

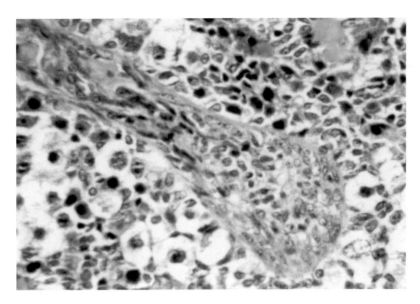

**Fig. 9-15** Gonadoblastoma, showing nests containing germ cells admixed with sex cord cells (note Call Exner–like structures (top right)) and intervening stroma with luteinized cells (top left). H&E, ×200.

## GONADOBLASTOMA

Patients are usually in their second decade[22] and have karyotype abnormalities, commonly gonadal dysgenesis (45X/46XY) or true hermaphroditism (46XY).

### GROSS

Tumors generally are unilateral and favor the right gonad, typically a streak. Size ranges from microscopic to 8 cm. Consistency varies from soft and fleshy to hard. Cut surface is solid yellow or brown with areas of calcification, sometimes extensive.

### HISTOLOGY

(Fig. 9-15). Germ cells and sex cord cells, in solid oval nests, are either intermixed or arranged as central germ cells and peripheral sex cord cells. Round eosinophilic structures, reminiscent of Call-Exner bodies, may be present. Stroma is scanty or abundantly fibrous, containing luteinized stromal cells and sometimes lymphocytes. Hyalinization and calcification are present. Germ cells resemble those in dysgerminomas. Sex cord cells are smaller and epithelial-like, with oval or elongated hyperchromatic nuclei. Mitotic activity occurs in germ cells.

## MIXED GERM CELL–SEX CORD–STROMAL TUMOR

Mixed germ cell–sex cord–stromal tumors are very rare. Patients are usually in their first decade and karyotypically normal (46XX).[23]

### GROSS

Tumors are usually unilateral, larger than gonadoblastomas, oval, and firm. Cut surface is solid or partly cystic and gray or yellow. Calcified areas are not present.

### HISTOLOGY

(Fig. 9-16). Germ cells and sex cord cells are admixed in trabeculae, small round nests, or solid masses.[24] Features that distinguish this tumor from gonadoblastoma include, in the mixed tumor, smaller nests of germ and sex cord cells, the latter usually of Sertoli versus granulosa cell variety; fewer luteinized stromal cells; brisker mitotic activity; and absence of hyalinization and calcification.

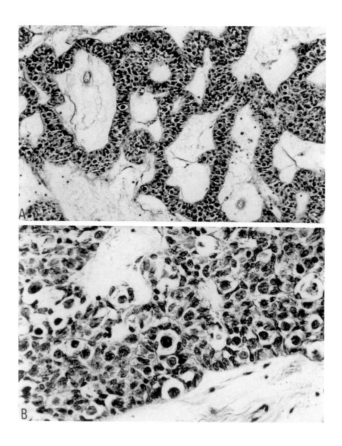

**Fig. 9-16** Mixed germ cell–sex cord–stromal tumor, showing columns containing germ cells (large pale) admixed with sex cord cells. H&E, (A) ×210, (B) ×525. (Courtesy Dr. A. Talerman, Rotterdam, Holland.)

## PLATES

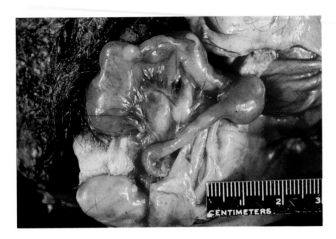

**Plate 9-1** Mature teratoma with recognizable segment of intestine

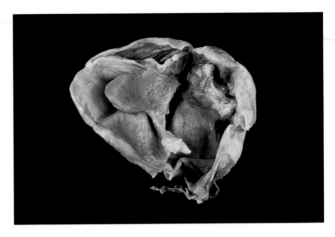

**Plate 9-2** Stroma ovarii showing recognizable thyroid tissue (brown)

# REFERENCES

1. Talerman A. Germ cell tumors of the ovary. In *Pathology of the Female Genital Tract,* 2d ed, Blaustein A, ed. New York, Springer-Verlag, 1982, pp 602–664.
2. Norris HJ, Jensen RD. Relative frequency of ovarian neoplasms in children and adolescents. *Cancer* 30:713–719, 1972.
3. Gordon A, Lipton D, Woodruff JD. Dysgerminoma: A review of 158 cases from the Emil Novak Ovarian Tumor Registry. *Obstet Gynecol* 58:497–504, 1981.
4. Asadourian LA, Taylor HB. Dysgerminoma. An analysis of 105 cases. *Obstet Gynecol* 33:370–379, 1969.
5. Meyer R. Pathology of some special ovarian tumors and their relation to sex characteristics. *Am J Obstet Gynecol* 22:697–713, 1931.
6. Mueller CW, Topkins P, Lapp WA. Dysgerminoma of the ovary. An analysis of 427 cases. *Am J Obstet Gynecol* 60:153–159, 1950.
7. Kurman RJ, Norris HJ. Endodermal sinus tumor of the ovary. A clinical and pathologic analysis of 71 cases. *Cancer* 38:2404–2419, 1976.
8. Teilum G. Endodermal sinus tumor. In *Special Tumors of Ovary and Testis and Related Extragonadal Lesions. Comparative Pathology and Histological Identification.* Philadelphia, Lippincott. 1976, pp 186–193.
9. Kurman RJ, Norris HJ. Embryonal carcinoma of the ovary. A clinico-pathologic entity distinct from endodermal sinus tumor resembling embryonal carcinoma of the adult testis. *Cancer* 38:2420–2433, 1976.
10. Pierce GB Jr, Midgley AR. The origin and function of human syncytiotrophoblastic giant cells. *Am J Pathol* 43:153–173, 1963.
11. Simard LC. Polyembryonic embryoma of the ovary of parthenogenetic origin. *Cancer* 10:215–223, 1957.
12. Beck JS, Fulmer HF, Lee ST. Solid malignant ovarian teratoma with "embryoid bodies" and trophoblastic differentiation. *J Pathol* 99:67–73, 1969.
13. Takeda A, Ishizuka T, Goto T, et al. Polyembryoma of ovary producing alpha-fetoprotein and HCG. Immunoperoxidase and electron microscopic study. *Cancer* 49:1878–1889, 1982.
14. Vance RP, Geisinger KR. Pure nongestational choriocarcinoma of the ovary. Report of a case. *Cancer* 56:2321–2325, 1985.
15. Woodruff JD, Protos P, Peterson WF. Ovarian teratomas. Relationship of histologic and ontogenic factors to prognosis. *Am J Obstet Gynecol* 102:702–715, 1968.
16. Brein JL, Neubecker RD. Ovarian malignancy in children with special reference to the germ cell tumors. *Ann NY Acad Sci* 142:658–674, 1967.
17. Norris HJ, Zirkin HJ, Benson WL. Immature (malignant) teratoma of the ovary. A clinical and pathologic study of 58 cases. *Cancer* 37:2359–2372, 1976.
18. Linder D, Power J. Further evidence for postmeiotic origin of teratomas in the human female. *Ann Hum Genetics* 34:21–30, 1970.
19. Peterson WF, Prevost EC, Edmunds FT, Huntley JM Jr, Morris FK. Benign cystic teratomas of the ovary. A clinico-statistical study of 1007 cases with review of the literature. *Am J Obstet Gynecol* 70:368–382, 1955.
20. Gusberg SB, Danforth DN. Clinical significance of struma ovarii. *Am J Obstet Gynecol* 48:537–542, 1944.
21. Scully RE. Recent progress in ovarian cancer. *Hum Pathol* 1:73–98, 1970.
22. Scully RE. Gonadoblastoma. A review of 74 cases. *Cancer* 25:1340–1356, 1970.
23. Talerman A. The pathology of gonadal neoplasms composed of germ cells and sex cord stroma derivations. *Pathol Res Pract* 170:24–38, 1980.
24. Talerman A. A distinctive gonadal neoplasm related to gonadoblastoma. *Cancer* 30:1219–1224, 1972.

# PART III. METASTATIC TUMORS

# 10

# Metastatic Ovarian Cancer

*Liane Deligdisch, M.D.*

The ovaries are the most common site for metastatic tumors in the female genital tract.[1] Approximately 15% of all ovarian malignant tumors are secondary. The most common metastatic tumors to the ovary originate in the gastrointestinal tract and in the breast. Tumors that originate in adjacent organs (uterus, fallopian tubes) may extend secondarily to the ovary; in many such cases with massive tumor involvement of multiple organs and adhesions, the primary site cannot be determined.

The frequency of metastatic ovarian cancer varies with the geographic location because of the difference in the prevalence of primary cancers. For example, in 1968, series from Japan and Hawaii reported a high incidence (40%) of gastric carcinomas metastatic to ovaries.[2] More recent series report a 6.2% incidence of metastatic gastric carcinoma to the ovary, in the U.S.[3] It seems that the patients with metastatic ovarian cancer are younger than those without ovarian involvement and that the spread of primary tumors to the ovaries is probably due to the more abundant vascularity in cycling ovaries.[4,5] Grossly, metastatic tumors to the ovary are mostly bilateral (approximately 20% of all bilateral ovarian tumors are metastatic) and often present as discrete nodules.

## METASTATIC GASTROINTESTINAL CANCERS

It is interesting to note that according to autopsy reports, gastric carcinoma is more frequently metastatic to the ovary than colonic carcinoma is, while in surgical reports, primary colonic carcinoma is more commonly metastatic to the ovary.[6] Both gastric and colonic carcinomas spread frequently to the ovaries, and ovarian metastases are usually found in patients younger than those without ovarian metastases.

## GASTRIC CARCINOMA

Gastric carcinoma (Krukenberg tumor) is characterized microscopically by mucin-filled signet ring cells diffusely infiltrating the ovarian stroma (Fig. 10-1). The primary origin is a gastric carcinoma, more often originating in the pyloric origin.

Grossly, Krukenberg tumors are round, often kidney-shaped (Plate 10-1), bosselated, firm whitish masses that can reach a large size; they are bilateral in over 80% of the cases. Rare gastric carcinomas metastatic to the ovary are not Krukenberg tumors and may be cystic. They have been frequently reported in young Japanese women.[2]

Histologically, the Krukenberg tumors reveal individual signet ring cells or clusters of such cells and occasional glands or tubular structures in an edematous (Fig. 10-2) or dense, storiform stroma. Blood and lymph vessels are often involved by tumor. Mucin stains are positive in most of the tumor cells (Plates 10-2 and 10-3). Adjacent stromal cells can show luteinization associated with hormone effect. Rare cases of Krukenberg tumors were considered primary ovarian because no other primary tumor could be identified.[7] Primary gastric carcinoma may be very small while the metastases to the ovaries are large. These tumors have a very poor prognosis.

**Fig. 10-1** Krukenberg tumor, showing clusters of tumor cells scattered in an edematous stroma. H&E, ×40.

## INTESTINAL CARCINOMA

Two to 10% of female patients with colonic carcinoma have metastases to the ovaries.[5] These metastases occur more often in patients older than those with Krukenberg tumors; the presenting symptom may be the ovarian tumor. In two-thirds of the cases, the ovarian tumors are large and bilateral. They are more often cystic than solid and often simulate ovarian tumors. Necrotic and mucinous areas are usually present (Plate 10-4). Histologically, the neoplastic cells are arranged in glands, or clusters, with mucin pools *(colloid carcinoma)* or exhibiting areas of necrosis surrounded by a rim of viable tumor (Fig. 10-3). Goblet cells are usually very numerous. The differential diagnosis with primary ovarian endometrioid carcinomas is discussed in Chap. 6.

Squamoid differentiation is absent in metastatic cancers (Fig. 10-4).

While most of the metastatic intestinal carcinomas arise in the colon, a number of cases originate from the appendix or small intestine.[8] Appendiceal carcinomas may be associated with primary ovarian mucinous tumors and with pseudomyxoma peritonei. In these cases, the histologic examination often reveals features of a borderline mucinous tumor.

## CARCINOID TUMORS

About 2% of metastatic ovarian tumors are primary carcinoids of small intestinal origin. Carcinoid syndrome is present in about 40% of cases.[9] Carcinoid tu-

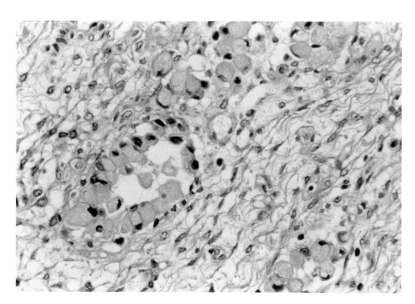

**Fig. 10-2** Krukenberg tumor, showing glandular structure and individual signet ring cells (top). H&E, ×400.

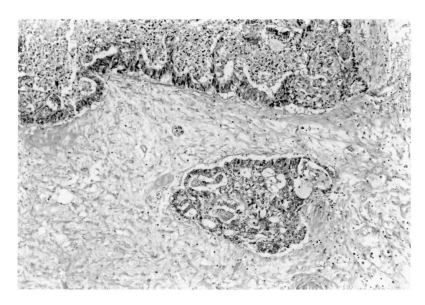

**Fig. 10-3** Metastatic colonic carcinoma. Necrotic zones are surrounded by viable adenocarcinoma in edematous ovarian stroma. H&E, ×100.

mors are bilateral, large, solid, and often yellowish, with smooth or bosselated surfaces showing occasional cystic degeneration or necrosis. Primary ovarian carcinoid tumors are usually associated with teratomas (germ cell tumors) and are unilateral. Histologically, both primary and metastatic ovarian carcinoids display insular (most frequently) (Fig. 10-5), trabecular (Fig. 10-6), or solid patterns. Special stains for neurosecretory granules are positive as are immunohistologic stains for chromogranin. The cells of carcinoid tumors typically have round nuclei with evenly distributed coarse chromatin and often contain argentaffin granules (Plate 10-5). The stroma may show a marked proliferation of spindle cells with hyalinization of the ground substance, or luteinized cells. The trabecular pattern of

carcinoid may resemble that of sex cord tumors, especially Sertoli–Leydig cell tumors. In carcinoid, these cords are larger and more regular. The acini of carcinoid tumors may resemble the Call-Exner bodies of granulosa cell tumors, which contain eosinophilic material that is mucin-negative.

A rather uncommon variant is the mucinous carcinoid tumor, or adenocarcinoid (Plate 10-6). They usually originate in the appendix.[10] Nests of goblet cells and round cavities filled with mucinous material are associated with various types of carcinoid cells (Figs. 10-7 and 10-8).

The primary source of carcinoid tumor is usually in the ileum but may occasionally be in the appendix, cecum, pancreas, colon, stomach, or lung.[9,11]

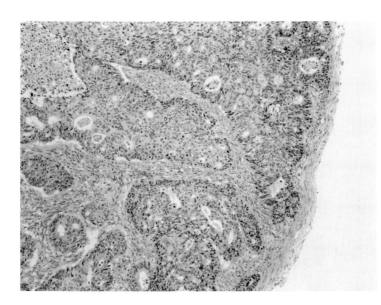

**Fig. 10-4** Metastatic colonic carcinoma. Ovary is infiltrated by moderately differentiated adenocarcinoma, somewhat reminiscent of endometrioid carcinoma. H&E, ×100.

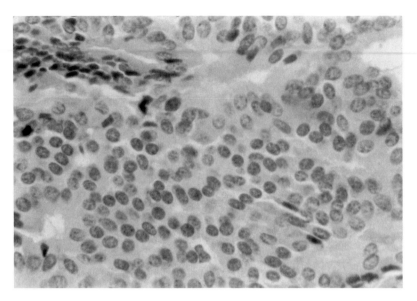

**Fig. 10-5** Metastatic carcinoid, insular type. H&E, ×100.

## METASTATIC BREAST CARCINOMAS

Examination of the ovaries removed to decrease estrogen levels in patients with widespread breast carcinoma has revealed the presence of metastatic tumor in 25 to almost 50% of the cases.[12] In the absence of clinical spread of the breast cancer, the incidence is much lower.[13] Grossly, these metastatic tumors were found to be more often bilateral. The ovaries are usually firm, nodular, whitish, and rarely cystic. The metastatic tumor is frequently a microscopic finding. Histologically, the tumor tissue resembles that of the primary breast tumor; tumor cells may be found in the highly vascularized theca or granulosa layer of the ovary in premenopausal, cycling patients, or in the ovarian stroma.

Lobular carcinoma (Fig. 10-9) spreads more often than ductal carcinoma (Fig. 10-10). The differential diagnosis with endometrioid ovarian and carcinoid tumors in particular may be difficult.

## SECONDARY TUMORS FROM UTERUS AND FALLOPIAN TUBES

Secondary involvement of the ovaries by tumors originating in adjacent organs, such as from the uterus or fallopian tubes, may occur by contiguous spread or by the lymphatic and vascular route (Plate 10-7). Squamous cell carcinoma of the cervix is uncommonly found to metastasize to the ovaries; in rare cases the

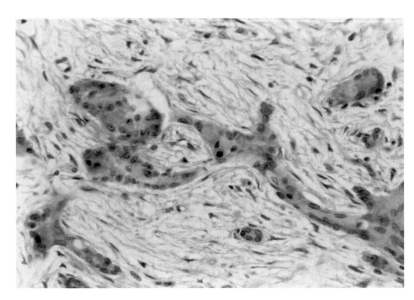

**Fig. 10-6** Metastatic carcinoid tumor, trabecular type. Nuclei show prominent coarse but evenly clumped chromatin. H&E, ×250.

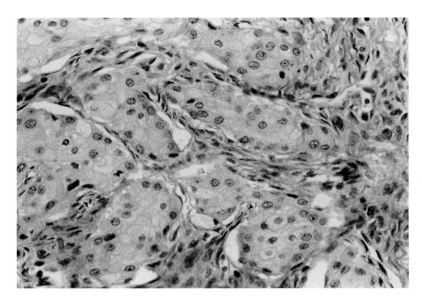

**Fig. 10-7** Metastatic mucinous carcinoid, showing mucinous adenocarcinoma and carcinoid-type nuclei. Primary tumor was in the appendix. H&E, ×250.

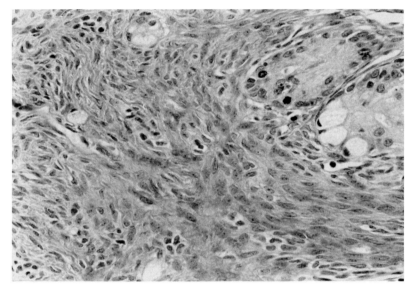

**Fig. 10-8** Metastatic mucinous carcinoid, showing hyperplastic ovarian stroma and mucinous adenocarcinoma with signet ring cells (right upper corner). H&E, ×250.

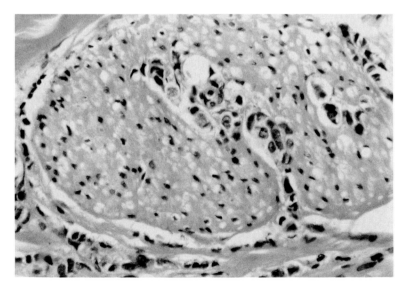

**Fig. 10-9** Metastatic breast carcinoma, lobular type, with perineural invasion. H&E, ×250.

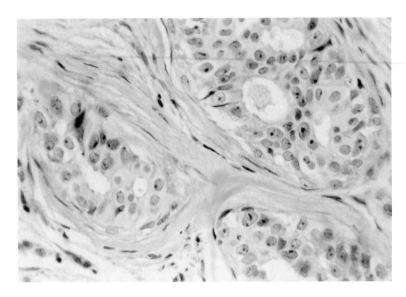

**Fig. 10-10** Metastatic breast carcinoma, ductal type. H&E, ×250.

primary neoplasm is a carcinoma in situ.[4] An unusual case of metastatic small cell carcinoma from the cervix presented with massive ovarian involvement (Plate 10-8). Histologically, the tumor tissue was similar to that seen in oat cell tumors of the lung and stained positively for chromogranin (Plate 10-9). Secondary involvement of the ovaries by uterine cancer is not unusual; it occurs by local spread, by contiguity via the fallopian tube, or by the lymphovascular route. The differential diagnosis between ovarian primary endometrioid carcinoma and metastatic endometrial carcinoma is discussed in Chap. 2. Metastatic tumor from the contralateral ovary is suggested by the finding of purely intravascular tumor tissue, in the absence of other tumor tissue. Metastatic tumors from primary fallopian tube sites are difficult to document and are of purely academic interest.

## METASTATIC OVARIAN TUMORS FROM OTHER PRIMARY SITES

### MALIGNANT MELANOMA

The primary site of these rare metastatic ovarian tumors to the ovaries is usually in the skin, occasionally in the choroid or elsewhere.[14] Ovarian metastases are present in 16% of women dying with malignant melanoma.[15] Metastatic malignant melanoma must be distinguished from the rare primary melanomas that arise from mature teratomas, occasionally associated with nevi found in mature skin tissue, which are usually unilateral and have a better prognosis. If no primary site can be identi-

fied at the time of the diagnosis, a regressed primary melanoma could possibly be the source of the ovarian metastasis.[16]

Grossly, metastatic malignant melanomas are usually bilateral, multinodular masses, variably pigmented (Plate 10-10), showing necrosis and cystic degeneration. Microscopically, they resemble primary malignant melanoma (Figs. 10-11 and 10-12). In the cases of amelanotic melanoma (Figs. 10-13 and 10-14) the differential diagnosis includes undifferentiated carcinoma, sarcoma, and dysgerminoma. Metastatic malignant melanomas resemble steroid cell tumors because of their abundant cytoplasm, prominent nucleoli, nuclear pleomorphism, and atypical mitotic activity as well as the immunohistochemical positive stain for S-100 protein; electron microscopic studies are diagnostic for malignant melanoma.

### MALIGNANT LYMPHOMA

The ovaries can be involved by disseminated malignant lymphoma, but are rarely the presenting site. Primary ovarian malignant lymphoma (Burkitt's lymphoma) is a specific type of malignant lymphoma found rarely outside the African continent; it has a multicentric origin and occurs mostly in children.

Because of the longer survival of patients with malignant lymphoma as a result of chemotherapy, the secondary involvement of the ovary became more common than the predominantly primary manifestation of this disorder.[5]

Grossly, both ovaries are usually involved; they may be enlarged or normal in size. Histologically, there is a diffuse infiltration by mostly poorly differentiated lym-

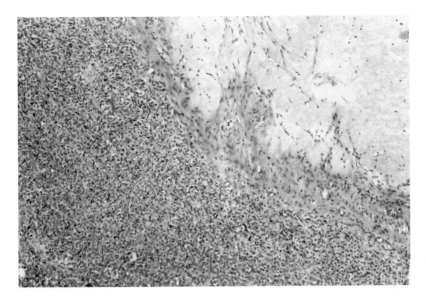

**Fig. 10-11** Metastatic malignant melanoma. The tumor surrounds ovarian corpus albicans. H&E, ×40.

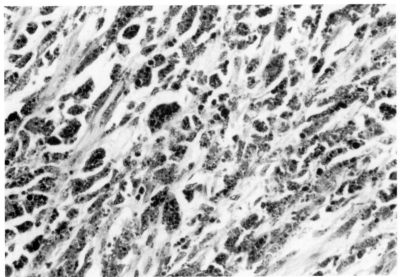

**Fig. 10-12** Pigmented metastatic malignant melanoma displaying melanin granules. Melanin Stain, ×100.

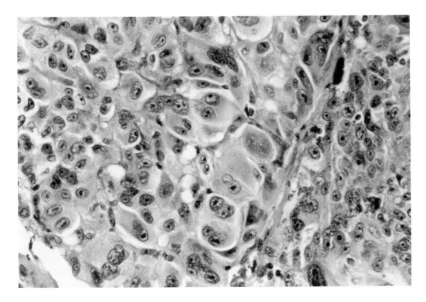

**Fig. 10-13** Amelanotic metastatic malignant melanoma. Note multinucleated giant cells and markedly prominent nucleoli. Abundant cytoplasm is somewhat reminiscent of lipid cell tumors. H&E, ×400.

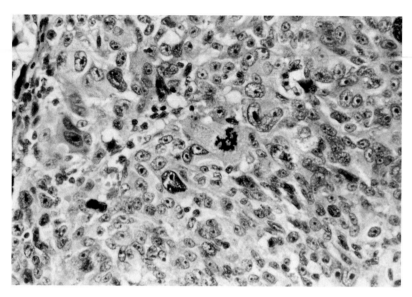

**Fig. 10-14** Metastatic malignant melanoma, showing marked nuclear pleomorphism and atypical mitosis (center). H&E, ×400.

phocytes, large or small cell types (Figs. 10-15 and 10-16).

## OAT CELL CARCINOMA

Oat cell carcinoma metastatic to the ovary is a rare occurrence. The primary site is in the lung or, exceptionally rare, in the uterine cervix (Fig. 10-17).

## CHORIOCARCINOMA

Choriocarcinoma of gestational origin, metastatic from a regressing trophoblastic tumor of uterus, is extremely rare (Fig. 10-18) and has to be distinguished from the ovarian nongestational choriocarcinoma, which is a primary germ cell tumor.

## RARE METASTATIC TUMORS

Tumors from the urinary tract may involve the ovaries secondarily by local extension or by the vascular route. Renal carcinomas may display histologic features somewhat similar to those of ovarian clear cell carcinomas; associated findings of endometrioid, squamoid features, ultrastructural characteristics, and, of course, the absence of lesions in the kidney confirm the primary nature of the ovarian clear cell carcinoma. Metastatic transitional cell carcinomas from the urinary bladder should be distinguished from the rare malignant Brenner tumors. Esophageal, gallbladder, pancreas, and thyroid tumors are infrequently found to metastasize to the ovary.

Sarcomas rarely metastasize to the ovary, neither do retroperitoneal tumors of neural origin. Metastatic neuroblastomas were reported in autopsy series.[17]

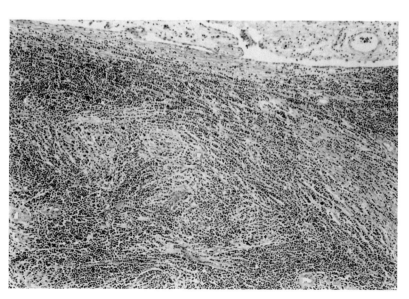

**Fig. 10-15** Malignant lymphoma with diffuse infiltration of the ovary (low power). Note periovarian adhesion (top). H&E, ×40.

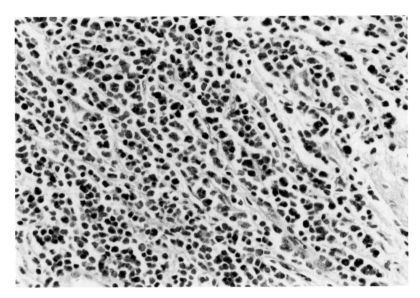

**Fig. 10-16** Malignant lymphoma, large cell type, same case in Fig. 10-15. H&E, ×400.

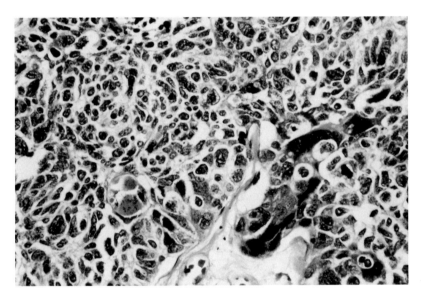

**Fig. 10-17** Metastatic oat cell carcinoma with bizarre giant multinucleated cells. H&E, ×400.

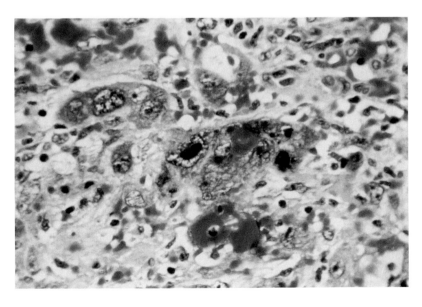

**Fig. 10-18** Metastatic choriocarcinoma exhibiting bizarre syncytiotrophoblastic cells. H&E, ×400.

**PLATES**

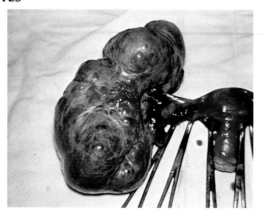

**Plate 10-1** Krukenberg tumor. Ovarian mass is solid, bulky, nodular, and reminiscent of a kidney (reniform). The tumor was bilateral.

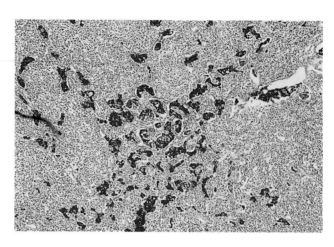

**Plate 10-2** Krukenberg tumor, specially stained for mucin. Numerous clusters of tumor cells, scattered in the ovarian stroma, stain positive for mucin. D-PAS stain, ×100.

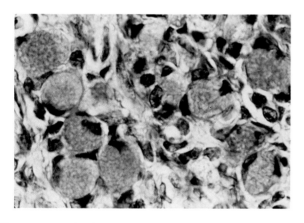

**Plate 10-3** Krukenberg tumor, specially stained for mucin. Signet ring cells display mucin-filled cytoplasm and peripheral nucleus. D-PAS, ×1000.

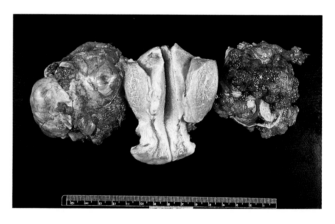

**Plate 10-4** Metastatic colonic carcinoma to ovaries, showing bilateral, bulky, partly cystic and partly solid tumors.

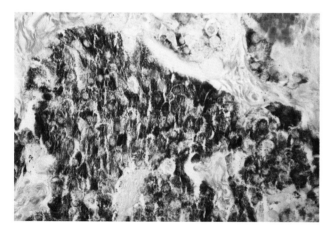

**Plate 10-5** Metastatic carcinoid tumor staining positive for neurosecretory granules.

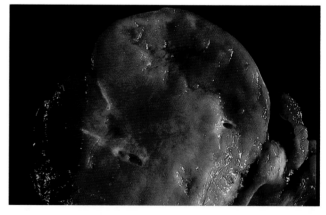

**Plate 10-6** Metastatic mucinous carcinoid. The tumor was bilateral.

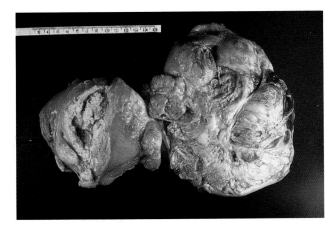

**Plate 10-7** Endometrial carcinoma with secondary involvement of the ovary.

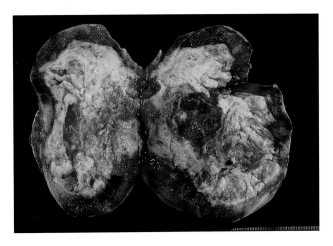

**Plate 10-8** Metastatic small cell carcinoma to ovary. Primary tumor was in the cervix. Ovarian tumor shows extensive necrosis.

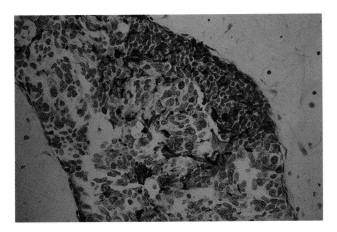

**Plate 10-9** Metastatic small cell carcinoma, exhibiting positive stain for chromogranin. ×400.

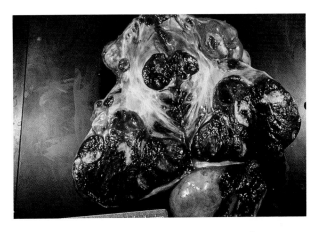

**Plate 10-10** Metastatic malignant melanoma. The patient had a primary malignant melanoma of the skin of the back. Ovarian tumor was soft, nodular, partly hemorrhagic, and partly pigmented.

## REFERENCES

1. Mazur MT, Hsueh S, Gasell DJ. Metastases to the female genital tract: Analysis of 325 cases. *Cancer* 53:1978–1984, 1984.
2. Hale RW. Krukenberg tumor of the ovaries: A review of 81 records. *Obstet Gynecol* 32:221–225, 1968.
3. Demopoulos RI, Touger L, Dubin N. Secondary ovarian carcinoma: A clinical and pathological evaluation. *Int J Gynecol Pathol* 6:166–175, 1987.
4. Young RH, Scully RE. Metastatic tumors of the ovary. In *Blaustein's Pathology of the Female Genital Tract,* 3d ed, Kurman, ed. New York, Springer-Verlag, pp 743–768, 1987.
5. Russell P, Ballantyne P. Tumors metastatic to the ovaries—Introduction. In *Surgical Pathology of the Ovaries.* Edinburgh, Churchill Livingstone, 1989, pp 474–482.
6. Webb MJ, Decker DG, Mussey E. Cancer metastatic to the ovary. Factors influencing survival. *Obstet Gynecol* 45:391–396, 1975.
7. Joshi VV. Primary Krukenberg tumor of the ovary. Review of literature and case report. *Cancer* 22:1199–1207, 1968.
8. Lash RH, Hart WR. Intestinal adenocarcinomas metastatic to the ovaries. A clinico-pathologic evaluation of 22 cases. *Am J Surg Pathol* 11:114–121, 1987.
9. Ulbright TM, Roth LM, Stehman FB. Secondary ovarian neoplasia. A clinico-pathologic study of 34 cases. *Hum Pathol* 16:28–34, 1984.
10. Hood IC, Jones BA, Watts JC. Mucinous carcinoid tumor of the appendix presenting as bilateral ovarian tumors. *Arch Pathol Lab Med* 110:336–340, 1986.
11. Robboy SJ, Scully RE, Norris HJ. Carcinoid metastatic to the ovary. A clinico-pathologic analysis of 35 cases. *Cancer* 33:798–811, 1974.
12. Puga FG, Gibbs CP, Williams TJ. Castrating operations associated with metastatic lesions of the breast. *Obstet Gynecol* 41:713–719, 1973.
13. Johansson H. Clinical aspects of metastatic ovarian cancer of extragenital origin. *Acta Obstet Gynecol Scand* 39:681–697, 1960.
14. Morrow CP, DiSaia PJ. Malignant melanoma of the female genitalia: A clinical analysis. *Obstet Gynecol Surv* 31:233–271, 1984.
15. Das Gupta T, Brasfield R. Metastatic melanoma. A clinico-pathologic study. *Cancer* 46:543–546, 1964.
16. Martinelli G, Tapparelli E, Merz R, Aldovini D, Zumiani G. Case of bilateral ovarian metastasis from regressed melanoma. *Eur J Gynaecol Oncol* 5:150–153, 1984.
17. Meyer WH, Yu GW, Milvenan ES, Jeffs RD, Kaizer H, Leventhal BG. Ovarian involvement in neuroblastoma. *Med Pediatr Oncol* 7:49–54, 1979.

# Appendix A

Histogenetic Classification of Ovarian Tumors (Modified from the 1973 WHO Classification)*

## PRIMARY OVARIAN TUMORS

I. COMMON EPITHELIAL TUMORS
   A. Serous—benign—cystadenoma and papillary cystadenoma
                    —adenofibroma and cystadenofibroma
        —of borderline malignancy (LMP)
        —malignant—serous papillary cystadenocarcinoma
                    —surface papillary peritoneal carcinoma
   B. Mucinous—benign—cystadenoma
                —of borderline malignancy (LMP)
                —malignant—cystadenocarcinoma
   C. Endometrioid—benign—adenofibroma and cystadenofibroma
                    —of borderline malignancy (LMP)
                    —endometrioid adenocarcinoma
                    —endometrioid stromal sarcoma
                    —malignant mixed mesodermal tumors
                            —homologous
                            —heterologous
   D. Clear cell—benign—adenofibroma
                —of borderline malignancy (LMP)
                —malignant—clear cell adenocarcinoma (mesonephroid)
   E. Brenner tumors—benign
                    —of borderline malignancy (LMP)
                    —malignant
   F. Undifferentiated carcinoma

II. SEX CORD STROMAL TUMORS
   A. Granulosa stromal cell tumor
      Granulosa cell tumor—adult type
                            —juvenile type
   B. Thecoma and fibroma
   C. Sclerosing stromal cell tumor
   D. Sertoli–Leydig cell tumors (androblastoma)
   E. Gynandroblastoma
   F. Sex cord tumor with annular tubules
   G. Unclassified

III. GERM CELL TUMORS
   A. Dysgerminoma
   B. Embryonal carcinoma (extraembryonic differentiation)
            —endodermal sinus tumor
            —choriocarcinoma (nongestational)
   C. Polyembryoma (embryonic differentiation)
   D. Teratoma
            —immature
            —mature (dermoid cyst)
            —specialized—struma ovarii
                    —strumal carcinoid
                    —carcinoid
   E. Mixed germ cell tumors
   F. Germ cell and sex cord stromal tumors
      Gonadoblastoma

*Serov SF, Scully RE, Sobin LH. Histological Typing of Ovarian Tumours. Geneva, World Health Organization a: p 37, b: pp 17–18, 1973.

# Appendix B

Carcinoma of the ovary: staging classification
using the FIGO nomenclature

| Stage | |
|---|---|
| Stage I | Growth limited to the ovaries. |
| Stage Ia | Growth limited to one ovary: no ascites; no tumor on the external surfaces; capsule intact. |
| Stage Ib | Growth limited to both ovaries; no ascites; no tumor on the external surfaces; capsules intact. |
| Stage Ic* | Tumor either stage 1a or stage 1b but with tumor on the surface of one or both ovaries; or with capsule ruptured; or with ascites present containing malignant cells or with positive peritoneal washings. |
| Stage IIa | Growth involving one or both ovaries with pelvic extension. |
| Stage IIa | Extension and/or metastases to the uterus and/or tubes. |
| Stage IIb | Extension to other pelvic tissues. |
| Stage IIc* | Tumor either stage IIa or stage IIb but with tumor on the surface of one or both ovaries; or with capsule(s) ruptured; or with ascites present containing malignant cells or with positive peritoneal washings. |
| Stage III | Tumor involving one or both ovaries with peritoneal implants outside the pelvis and/or positive retroperitoneal or inguinal nodes; superficial liver metastasis equals stage III; tumor limited to the true pelvis but with histologically verified malignant extension to small bowel or omentum. |
| Stage IIIa | Tumor grossly limited to the true pelvis with negative nodes but with histologically confirmed microscopic seeding of abdominal peritoneal surfaces. |
| Stage IIIb | Tumor of one or both ovaries: histologically confirmed implants of abdominal peritoneal surfaces, none exceeding 2 cm in diameter; nodes negative. |
| Stage IIIc | Abdominal implants 2 cm in diameter and/or positive retroperitoneal or inguinal nodes. |
| Stage IV | Growth involving one or both ovaries with distant metastasis; pleural effusion present, there must be positive cytologic test results to allot a case to stage IV; parenchymal liver metastasis equals stage IV. |

SOURCE: Oncology Committee of the International Federation of Gynecology and Obstetrics: Changes in Definitions of Clinical Staging for Carcinoma of the Cervix and Ovary: International Federation of Gynecology and Obstetrics *Am J Obstet Gynecol* 156:263–264, 1987. *Clinical Gynecologic Oncology*, DiSaia PJ, Creasman WT, eds. St. Louis, Mosby, 1989, p 336.

# Index